Annual Review of Hydrocephalus
Volume 5   1987

Editors:

Satoshi Matsumoto, M.D.
Kobe University, School of Medicine, Kobe
Editor-in-Chief

Kiyoshi Sato, M.D.
Juntendo University, School of Medicine, Tokyo
Norihiko Tamaki, M.D.
Kobe University, School of Medicine, Kobe
Shizuo Oi, M.D.
Kobe University, School of Medicine, Kobe

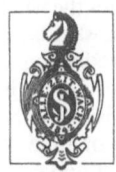

Springer-Verlag Berlin Heidelberg GmbH

This work is published originally by Neuron Publishing Co.

ISBN 978-3-662-11151-2   ISBN 978-3-662-11149-9 (eBook)
DOI 10.1007/978-3-662-11149-9

Softcover reprint of the hardcover 1st edition 1989

Originally published by Springer-Verlag Berlin Heidelberg New York in 1989.

Annual Review of Hydrocephalus

Editors:

Satoshi Matsumoto, M. D.
Kobe University, School of Medicine, Kobe
Editor-in-Chief

Kiyoshi Sato, M. D.
Juntendo University, School of Medicine, Tokyo
Norihiko Tamaki, M. D.
Kobe University, School of Medicine, Kobe
Shizuo Oi, M. D.
Kobe University, School of Medicine, Kobe

Volume 5   1987

ISBN 978-3-662-11151-2   ISBN 978-3-662-11149-9 (eBook)
DOI 10.1007/978-3-662-11149-9

Published by
NEURON Publishing Co.
21–19, Higashi-Gotanda 5-chome
Shinagawa-ku, Tokyo 141, Japan

PREFACE

This volume contains 110 representative works on hydrocephalus which are collected from 26 listed journals and books in the field of neuroscience published in 1986.

We express our sincere thanks to all authors, listed publishers and editorial boards for their cooperation and permission on this publication.

It is our pleasure if this book will provide you with an up-to-date review of the works on hydrocephalus.

The editors

ACKNOWLEDGMENT

Greatful acknowledgments for permission to reproduce copyright material are made to the editors and the publishers listed below:

Acta Cytologica: The International Academy of Cytology

Acta Neurochirurgica: Springer-Verlag

Acta Neurochirurgica: Springer-Verlag, Wein

Acta Neurologica Scandinavica: Munksgaard International Publishers Ltd.

Acta Neuropathologica: Springer-Verlag, Heidelberg

American Journal of Neuroradiology (AJNR): American Roentgen Ray Society

Annals of Neurology: American Neurological Association

Annual Report of the Research Committee of "Hydrocephalus," The Ministry of Health and Welfare of Japan, 1986: Neuron Publishing Co.

Archives of Neurology: American Medical Association

Brain and Development: (Official Journal of The Japanese Society of Child Neurology)

British Journal of Obstetrics and Gynaecology: Blackwell Scientific Publications Ltd.

Child's Nervous System: Springer-Verlag, Berlin

CT Kenkyu/Progress in Computerized Tomography: Neuron Publishing Co.

Journal of Computer Assisted Tomography: Raven Press, New York

Journal of Neurology, Neurosurgery and Psychiatry: British Medical Journal

Journal of Neurosurgery: The American Association of Neurological Surgeons

Journal of Pediatric Neurosciences: Springer-Verlag, Heidelberg

Journal of Pediatric Surgery: Grune & Stratton, Inc.

Journal of Ultrasound in Medicine: American Institute of Ultrasound in Medicine

Neuropediatrics: Hippokrates Verlag GmbH

Neurosurgery: The Congress of Neurological Surgeons, Inc.

No to Hattatsu: (Official Journal of the Japanese Society of Child Neurology) Shindan to
                 Chiryo Sha

No to Shinkei/Brain & Nerve: Igaku Shoin

Noshinkei Geka/Neurological Surgery: Igaku Shoin

Shoni no Noshinkei/Nervous System in Children: Neuron Publishing Co.

The Canadian Journal of Neurological Sciences: University Calgary Press

CONTENTS

I) EXPERIMENTAL & BASIC STUDIES

HYDROCEPHALUS MODELS

PATHOLOGY

PHYSIOLOGY

METABOLISM·CHEMISTRY

II) PATHOPHYSIOLOGY

HYDRODYNAMICS

INTRACRANIAL PRESSURE

ETIOPATHOGENESIS

III) SYMPTOMATOLOGY

IV) DIAGNOSTIC PROCEDURES

CT & CT CISTERNOGRAPHY

NMR·POSITRON CT

SHUNT FUNCTION (TEST)

SHUNT COMPLICATIONS

VI) FOLLOW-UP & LONG-TERM RESULT

VII) CLASSIFICATION OF HYDROCEPHALUS

CONGENITAL

CRANIUM BIFIDUM AND SPINA BIFIDA

HOLOPROSENCEPHALY

CONGENITAL CYST

NORMAL PRESSURE HYDROCEPHALUS

INDEX

I) Experimental and Basic Studies

Hydrocephalus Models
Pathology
Physiology
Metabolism · Chemistry

Ultrastructural Morphology of the Olfactory Pathway for Cerebrospinal Fluid Drainage in the Rabbit

Stephanie S. ERLICH, J. Gordon McComb, Shigeyo HYMAN, and Martin H. WEISS

Department of Neurological Surgery, University of Southern California School of Medicine; and Division of Neurosurgery, Children's Hospital of Los Angeles, Los Angeles, California, USA

Previous physiological studies indicate that the olfactory region serves as a major pathway for cerebrospinal fluid (CSF) drainage into the lymphatic system. The present study was undertaken to determine the ultrastructural characteristics of this egress route. New Zealand White rabbits received a single bolus injection of the tracer ferritin (MW 400,000) into both lateral ventricles in such a manner as not to raise the intraventricular pressure above the normal level. The animals were sacrificed via intracardiac perfusion of fixative between less than 12 minutes and 4 hours following injection. The cribriform region was removed *en bloc*, decalcified, sectioned coronally, and prepared for light and electron microscopic examination.

The arachnoid, dura, and periosteum surrounding the fila olfactoria passing through the cribriform plate merge together and form the perineurium, which consists of multiple layers of loosely overlapping cells with widely separated junctions and few vesicles. The perineurium surrounding the olfactory filaments at the superficial submucosal level is only one cell thick. The subarachnoid space freely communicates with the perineural space surrounding each filament. No morphological barrier between the perineural space and the loose submucosal connective tissue was identified. Whether or not the perineurium was multi- or single-layered, ferritin was noted in abundance between the loosely overlapping perineural cells and in the submucosal connective tissue. The distribution of ferritin at 12 minutes was similar to that at 4 hours; however, the quantity of ferritin was increased at 4 hours. These results indicate that no significant barrier to CSF drainage is present at the rabbit cribriform region and that CSF reaches the submucosal region rapidly via open pathways. (J Neurosurg 64: 466–473, 1986)

Key words: Cerebrospinal fluid absorption, Cribriform plate, Ultrastructural study, Olfactory tract, Rabbit

Aqueductal Lesions in 6-aminonicotinamide-treated Suckling Mice

Hisashi Aikawa,[1,2] Shigeichi Kobayashsi,[2] and Kinuko Suzuki[2]

[1]Division of Ultrastructural Research, National Institute of Neuroscience, Tokyo, Japan; and [2]Department of Pathology and Neuroscience, Albert Einstein College of Medicine, Bronx, New York, USA

Suckling mice which received a single intraperitoneal injection of 6-aminonicotinamide on the 5th postnatal day, consistently developed hydrocephalus. During the early stages of hydrocephalus (7–9 days after injection), aqueductal lesions were characterized by edematous ependymal and subependymal cells, and spongy changes in the periaqueductal area, which resulted in aqueduct stenosis. Later stages (after 20 days post-injection) showed that these edematous changes totally subsided, leaving an obliterated aqueduct which was similar to that of human congenital hydrocephalus. At the completely obliterated area, ultrastructural investigation disclosed a normal-looking neuropil but no aqueductal lumen. In the remaining ependymal cells, increased intermediate filaments and lipid droplets occurred. These data suggest that acute ependymal cell degeneration during the perinatal period may result in the profile of aqueduct "agensis" in human congenital hydrocephalus.

(Acta Neuropathol 71: 243–250, 1986)

Key words: 6-Aminonicotinamide, Aqueduct "agenesis," Ependymal cell, Hydrocephalus, Suckling mice

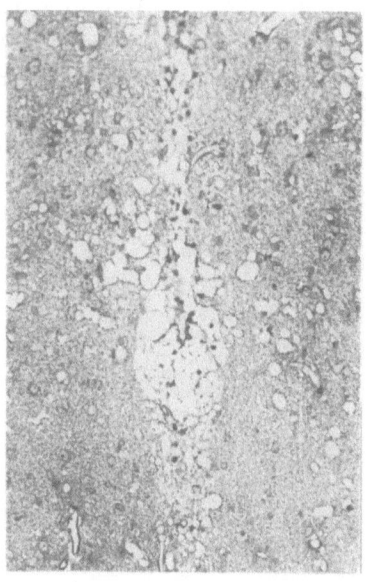

Figure. An aqueductal lesion in a 6-AN-treated mice. On Day 7 postinjection of 6-AN, the aqueduct is obliterated with vacuolated ependymal cells and subependymal glial cells. Spongy changes in the periaqueductal gray matter are also prominent.
One-micrometer Epon Section. Toluidin blue stain. ×240

Characteristics of Brain Tissue Damage in Kaolin-induced Infantile Rat Hydrocephalus

Tohru Okuyama,[1] Kazuo Hashi,[1] Tadashi Okada,[1] and Satoshi Sasaki[2]

[1]Department of Neurosurgery, Sapporo Medical College, Sapporo; and [2]Department of Veterinary Physiology, Obihiro University of Agriculture and Veterinary Medicine, Obihiro, Japan

Experimental of hydrocephalus was induced by an intracisternal injection of 4% or 40% kaolin suspension in 2 days old Wistar rats. They were examined histologically and microangiographically 2 weeks after the injection of kaolin.

Hydrocephalic rats were classified into 2 groups, severe hydrocephalic group A and mild hydrocephalic group B. In group A, a marked enlargement of the entire ventricular system with a thinning of the cerebral mantle was observed. On the other hand, the dilatation of the fourth ventricle was more pronounced compared with the other ventricles in group B. In group A, a spongy appearance of brain tissue was observed in the periventricular white

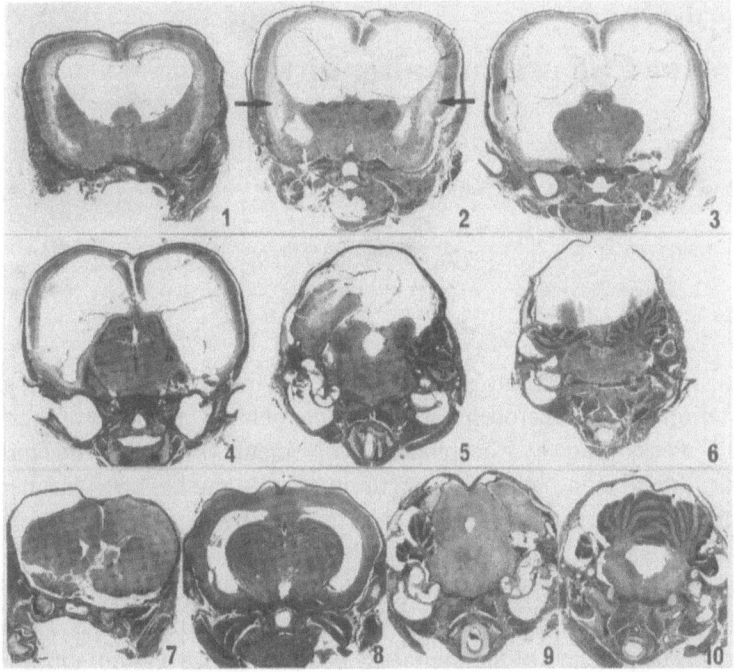

Figures 1–6. Sixteen-day-old rat with severe hydrocephalus (group A). Marked enlargement of Sylvian aqueduct and lateral ventricles. Edematous white matter with intracerebral cavity (*arrows*). HE, ×3.8

Figures 7–10. Seventeen-day-old rat with mild hydrocephalus (group B). Enlargement of the fourth ventricle is more pronounced compared with the other ventricles. HE, ×3.8

matter accompanied with an intracerebral cavity. In these edematous areas, the lack of carbon black perfusion was apparent indicating an occurrence of microcirculatory disturbances. These microcirculatory disturbances and mechanical compression to the cerebral parenchyma may produce defective brain tissue (intracerebral cavity formation). The ependymal cell walls and subependymal glial cell layers were well preserved in spite of the damaged periventricular white matter.

In group A, kaolin was present in the fourth ventricle and Sylvian aqueduct. Subependymal gliosis containing macrophages and newly produced blood vessels were observed in the region between the periventricular brain tissue and kaolin granules. These findings indicate that kaolin may produce changes in the ependymal cell and cerebral parenchyma as well as fibrosis and meningitis in the subarachnoid space.   (Brain and Nerve 38: 69–74, 1986)

Key words: Hydrocephalus, Infantile rat, Kaolin, Morphology, Intracerebral cavity

Histogenetic Disorders of the Cerebral Cortex Caused by Prenatal ^{60}Co gamma-Irradiation and Manifestation of Hydrocephalus:
Changes of the CSF pressure after birth

Yoshiro Kameyama, Shoko Kimura, and Yoshihiro Fukui

The Research Institute of Environmental Medicine, Nagoya University, Nagoya, Japan

In the previous paper, the authors reported that mice irradiated with Co-60 gamma-rays on day 13 of gestation showed microcephaly at the time of birth, and most of them who survived more than 2 weeks had hydrocephalic involvement. Prior to the manifestation of hydrocephalus, blood congestion in the brain mantle, periventricular hemorrhage and subsequent tissue destruction were detected in high frequency.

The present study was designated to examine the relationship between the change of CSF pressure and the manifestation of hydrocephalus in mice irradiated on the day 13 of gestation. The CSF pressure was measured at the cisterna magna in mice from one day to 40 days after birth. The pressure of the prenatally irradiated mice was not different from that of the non-treated normal mice until 12 days after birth. In this normal pressure periods, the irradiated mice had been already involved with tissue destructive changes of the brain mantle and enlargement of the lateral ventricles, which condition was regarded as hydrocephalus ex vacuo. Around 14 days after birth, the pressure of the irradiated mice began to increase concurrently with an external appearance of vaulted skull. This finding indicated that microhydrocephalus of ex vacuo in nature transformed to high-pressure hydrocephalus at the time of brain growth spurt.

(Annual Report of the Research Committee of "Hydrocephalus," The Ministry of Health and Welfare of Japan, 1986: 65–70, 1987)

Key words: CSF pressure, Experimental hydrocephalus, Co-60 gamma-irradiation

Growth Pattern of the Telencephalic Choroid Plexus of Rat Embryo

Mitsunori YAMADA,[1] Yasuji YOSHIDA,[2] Koichi WAKABAYASHI,[1] and Fusahiro IKUTA[1]

Departments of [1]Pathology and [2]Neuropathology, Brain Research Institute, Niigata University, Niigata, Japan

We studied the morphological development and cytogenesis of the telencephalic choroid plexus in the rat from embryonic day 13 (E13) to 20. Cell proliferation was investigated with bromodeoxyuridine (BrdU), an analogue of thymidine. Based on the results of preliminary studies on the cytotoxic effects of BrdU and the appropriate dose for immunohistochemical detection, 20 mg/kg of BrdU was injected intraperitoneally to each pregnant rat. Fetuses were removed respectively 1 and 4 hours after the injection, and BrdU-incorporated nuclei were demonstrated by the avidine-biotin peroxidase complex method.

On E14, small bulges were formed at the medial wall of the cerebral hemispheres. The covering epithelium was pseudostratified and had many BrdU-positive nuclei. On E15, a fold-like anlage of the choroid plexus developed. Although near to the root of the fold the epithelium was still pseudostratified, more distally it was transformed into single-layered, and BrdU-positive epithelial cells became sparse around the apex. After E16, as the development progressed, most of the epithelium became simple columnar, with the pseudostratified epithelium remained at the junction with the neural epithelium. In these stages, BrdU-positive epithelial cells were largely restricted to the root of the plexus, but a few were also observed at the apex or the trunk. In the choroid plexus stroma, on the other hand, many BrdU-positive cells were distributed in a diffuse pattern from the root to the apex, throughout the development.

These results indicate that rapid proliferation of choroidal epithelium occurs at the root of the plexus, while meningovascular tissue proliferates diffusely in the plexus stroma. In addition, the existence of some BrdU-positive epithelial cells in the trunk or apex of the plexus at the late developing stages strongly suggests that a low rate of epithelial proliferation occurs even at these portions until perinatal stage at least.

(Annual Report of the Research Committee of "Hydrocephalus," The Ministry of Health and Welfare of Japan, 1986: 15–22, 1987)

Key words: Telencephalic choroid plexus, Cytogenesis, Bromodeoxyuridine, Development, Rat

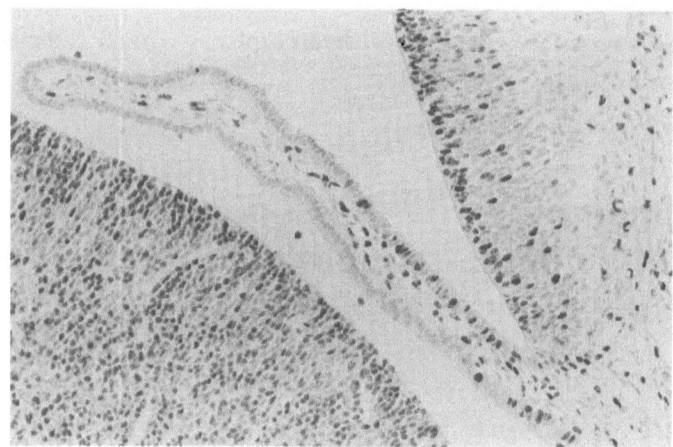

Figure. Telencephalic choroid plexus in rat fetus on embryonic day 16. BrdU-positive epithelial cells are largely restricted to the root of the plexus. Four hours after the BrdU injection. BrdU immunohistochemistry. ×200

Pathogenesis of Cerebral Tissue Damage on Experimental Hydrocephalus:
Ultrastructural changes in kaolin induced rat hydrocephalus

Takashi Tsubokawa, Mitsusuke Miyagami, and Tadashi Shibuya

Department of Neurological Surgery, Nihon University School of Medicine, Tokyo, Japan

In order to clarify the pathogenesis of cerebral tissue damage on the kaolin-induced rat hydrocephalus, morphological evaluation was performed on the acute and chronic stage of hydrocephalus at 1 to 10 weeks after injection of kaolin in to the cisternal magna of 20 wistar rats with both light and electron microscopic studies.

More than 70% of the rats injected kaolin revealed moderate or marked ventricular dilatation and in chronic stage the ventricles were more dilated than in acute stage. It was found apparently that hydrocephalic rats had irregularly depressed cillia with fewer microvilli and the clefts between ependymal cells on the surface of lateral ventricles especially more than 4 weeks after kaolin injection in scanning electron microscopic study.

Histologically more extensive spongy state was observed in the periventricular tissues of acute hydrocephalic rats than in that of chronic hydrocephalus. The ultrastructural changes of hydrocephalic rats were found distinctly in the neuron and the glia cells of subependymal layer and white matter within 100 μm from the ventricular wall surface. The extracellular spaces due to edema were enlarged and decreased electron density in acute stage of them. Intracellular edema was seen in the cytoplasm of the neuronal processes and glia cells in both acute and chronic stage of hydrocephalic rats. The degenerative changes having the abnormal electron density, vacuole or lamellar structure formation and decreasement or the destruction of neurotubulus were found in the cytoplasm of some dendrites and axons in the periventricular tissues of chronic hydrocephalic rats more than 4 weeks after injection of kaolin.

It was suggested that cerebral tissue damages of hydrocephalic rats were found as the degenerative changes and intracellular edema of the neuronal processes and glia cells in periventricular tissues in chronic stage of them.

(Annual Report of the Research Committee of "Hydrocephalus," The Ministry of Health and Welfare of Japan, 1986: 51–56, 1987)

Key words: Experimental hydrocephalus, Electron microscopy, Kaolin, Brain edema, Lateral ventricle

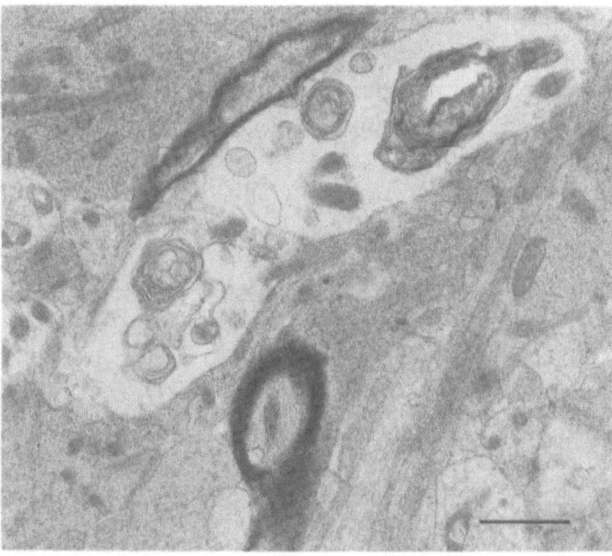

Figure. This demonstrates neuronal processes with degenerative change having decrease of electron density, vacuole, and remarkable multilamellar body in periventricular tissue of chronic hydrocephalic rat at 4 weeks after kaolin injection.

Morphological Findings of Postshunt Slit-ventricle in Experimental Canine Hydrocephalus:
Aspects of causative factors of isolated ventricles and slit-ventricle syndrome

Shizuo Oi[1] and Satoshi Matsumoto[2]

Department of Neurosurgery, [1]National Kagawa Children's Hospital, Zentsuji, Kagawa; and [2]Kobe University School of Medicine, Kobe, Japan

The progressive status of slit-ventricle and its associated pathology may be severe, occasionally resulting in the slit-ventricle syndrome or irreversible morphological changes in the brain and CSF pathways. To analyze the morphological changes of slit-ventricles critically, comparing the human form with canine hydrocephalus, 19 dogs had kaolin injected into the cisterna magna to produce hydrocephalus. The model of slit-ventricle was created by a low pressure arrangement (external ventricular drainage with extreme siphon effect). The gross morphological appearance showed thickening of the white matter, enlarged cortical vessels, and slit-ventricles. The brain parenchyma changes were observed as disorganized, with partially stripped-off ependymal lining, remarkable gliotic scar tissue in the subependymal areas and adjacent white matter, and widely opened Virchow-Robin spaces. These seem to be responsible for the decreased intracranial compliance and isolation of the CSF pathways.   (Child's Nerv Syst 2: 179–184, 1986)

Key words: Slit-ventricle, Morphological changes, Experimental canine hydrocephalus, Isolated ventricles, Slit-ventricle syndrome

Table.   Morphological change in experimental hydrocephalus

	Hydrocephalus (2 months after kaolin injection)	Unilaterally overdrained brain (after 1 week overdrainage from left lateral ventricle)	
		Right cerebral hemisphere with a dilated lateral ventricle	Left cerebral hemisphere with a slit like ventricle
Ependymal layer	Flattened cells, interrupted lining	Normalized lining	Partially interrupted lining
Subependymal layer	Spongy swelling, expanded extracellular space, loss of astrocytes, cerebrospinal fluid edema	Less prominent findings of cerebrospinal fluid edema	Narrow extracellular space
White matter			Disorganized layer Prominent gliosis
Cerebral cortex	No remarkable changes	No remarkable changes	No remarkable changes
Virchow-Robin space	Collapsed	Narrow	Widely open
Vascular beds	Collapsed	Normalized	Dilated

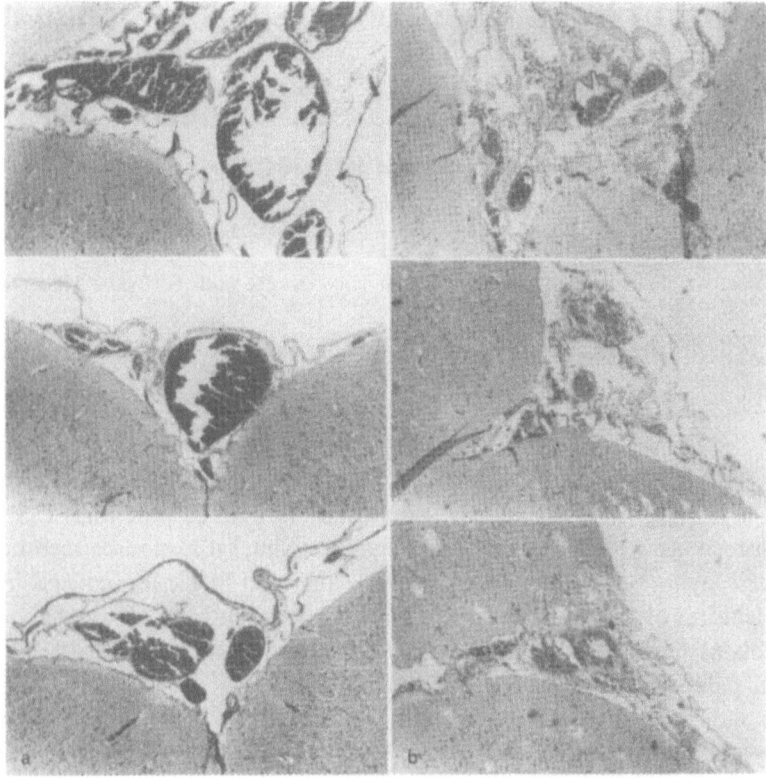

Figure 1. Vascular beds of cortical vessels: **a)** slit-ventricle, **b)** hydrocephalus. Note remarkable expansion in the slit-ventricle side.

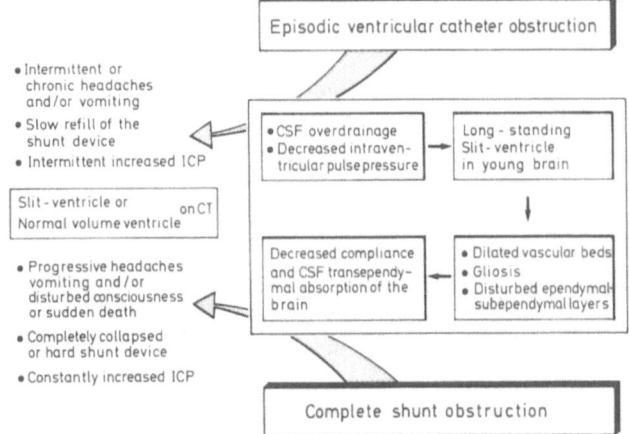

Figure 2. Possible pathogenesis of "slit-ventricle syndrome" or "normal volume hydrocephalus" [13].

Mechanisms of Impairment of Cerebral Function in Hydrocephalus (Part 4):
Neurophysiological evaluation of axonal conduction, synaptic transmission and postsynaptic integrations

Takashi Tsubokawa, Yoichi Katayama, Tatsuro Kawamata, and Teruyasu Hirayama

Department of Neurological Surgery, Nihon University School of Medicine, Tokyo, Japan

In order to clarify the functional background underlying the neurologic deficits in chronic hydrocephalus, change in short latency somatosensory evoked potentials (SSEP), cortico-spinal direct responses (D-response), and Schaffer collateral responses recorded from CAl pyramidal cell layers of the hippocampus were analyzed in kaolin-induced hydrocephalic rats. Other features of this rat model of chronic hydrocephalus were evaluated on the basis of measurements of the intracranial pressure, Na-fluorescein migration from the ventricle to the cerebral parenchyma and bihavioral changes.

The results indicated that (1) the central conduction time calculated from SSEP was substantially unaffected (*Figure 1*), (2) the latency of D-response was unchanged, (3) the conduction velocity of the Schaffer collateral was unchanged, (4) the threshold to elicit

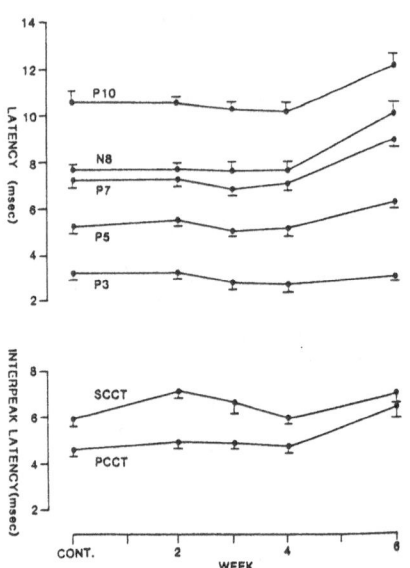

Figure 1. Time-curves of the latencies of SSEPs (*upper*), the primary central conduction time (PCCT) and the secondary central conduction time (SCCT) (*lower*) record in hydrocephalic rats.

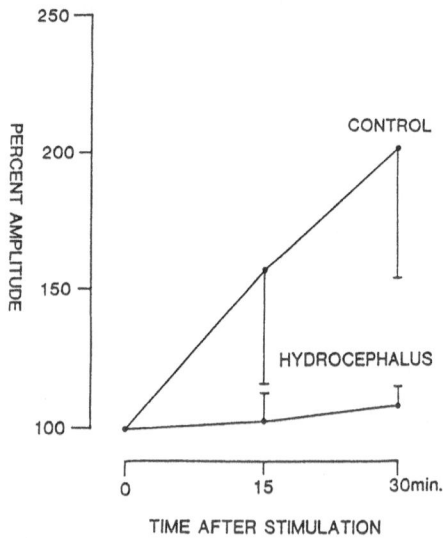

Figure 2. The changes of long-term potentiation in the hippocampus of hydrocephalic rats.

population spikes was decreased, (5) the paired-pulse facilitation of EPSP tended to increase, (6) the paired-pulse inhibition of population spikes was unchanged and (7) long-term potentiation (LTP) of the population spikes was clearly attenuated in the hydrocephalic rats (*Figure 2*). The deficits seen in the long-term potentiation were less pronounced in rats which underwent kaolin injection but did not develop hydrocephalus. The above findings suggest that disturbance of the postsynaptic integration processes, rather than axonal conduction or synaptic transmission, is more important for the induction of neurologic deficits in chronic hydrocephalus.

Many previous studies have demonstrated that the phenomenon of LTP seen in the hippocampus is related to behavioral learning. Therefore the fact of the impaired LTP in chronic hydrocephalus is very much interesting on thinking about mechanisms of recent memory disturbance which is one of the major symptoms of chronic hydrocephalus in humans. Concerning the morphological changes attributed to the induction of neurologic deficits in chronic hydrocephalus, many of previous observations have attended to interstitial edema or axonal degeneration in white matter. On this study, however, importance of the impairment of dendrites is found as dying-back phenomenon by EMS observation, which is completely coincidence with alteration of LTP.

(Annual Report of the Research Committee of "Hydrocephalus," The Ministry of Health and Welfare of Japan, 1986: 57–63, 1987)

Key words: Somatosensory evoked potential (SEP), Corticospinal direct response, Long-term potentiation (LTP), Dendrite damage, Hydrocephalus, Rats

Analysis of Difficult Cases on the Treatment of Hydrocephalic Children

Tetsuro Miwa and Hiroshi Ito

Department of Neurosurgery, Tokyo Medical College, Tokyo, Japan

Generally, the non-tumorous hydrocephalus in childhood often has been very successfully treated. However, the prognosis of some cases is poor even when the shunting procedure has been performed.

Disability and death due to hydrocephalus are very serious problem, so we have attempted to obtain a new interpretation of the influence factor upon the prognosis and we studied analyses of difficult cases after the operative treatment.

In the period between 1972 and 1985 at the Department of Neurosurgery, Tokyo Medical College Hospital, surgical procedure was carried out in 72 cases of child hydrocephalus. 43 cases survived and 24 cases died. We have tried to evaluate hydrocephalus throuth the investigation of morphological analyses of the head and brain, CSF pressure study and chemical analysis of the metabolic substances in CSF.

From our results, in the cases which showed poor prognosis, abnormal decrease rate compared to standard rate and less than 12mm thickness of the cerebral mantle were recognized within the first three months of life. In addition, poor cases showed monophasic low amplitude waves in the pressure study of intraventricular CSF and abnormal high values of HVA, 5-HIAA in CSF (*Figure*). Fatty acid values, which were remarkably unstable during the postoperative period, tended to lead to poor prognosis.

In 15 cases, death occurred more than three years after the operation for hydrocephalus. Six out of 15 cases died suddenly in spite of the shunt functioning well and these cases presented the so-called "hydrocephalic crisis."

Autopsy cases demonstrated the small, shallow posterior cranial fossa and an anatomical abnormal structure play roles in developing into an abortive form of craniocerebral disproportion. These pathological changes are easily affected by elevation of the supratentorial CSF pressure.

The outcome was reviewed in six cases with severe hydrocephalus who were diagnosed during the perinatal period. The irremediable cerebral malformation affected on prognosis. Each case must be considered individually, and further consideration is necessary before we come to our final decision.

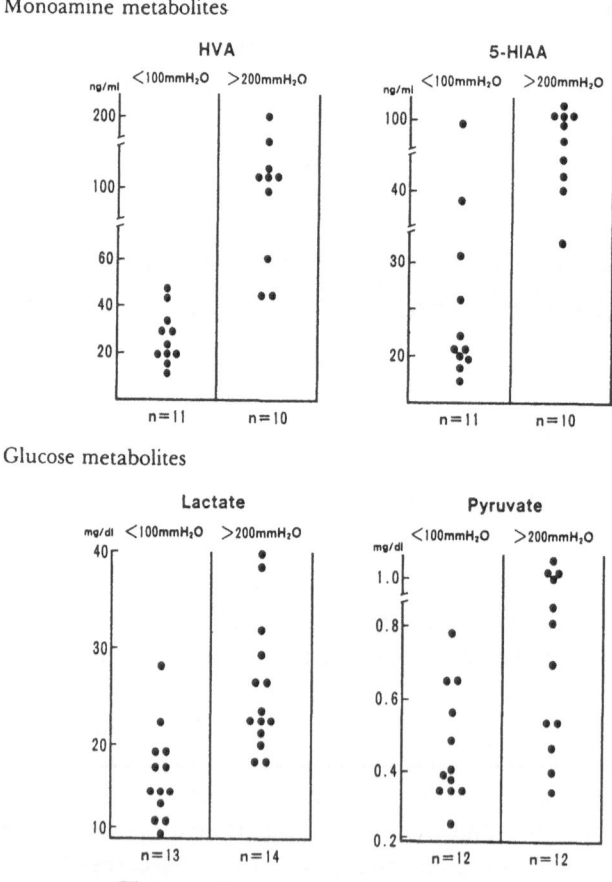

Figure. Various metabolites in CSF.

On the above results, we must take a continuous attitude toward the problems related to extraction of difficult cases on the treatment of hydrocephalic children.

(Annual Report of the Reseach Committee of "Hydrocephalus," The Ministy of Health and Welfare of Japan, 1986: 133–141, 1987)

Key words: Hydrocephalus, Cerebrospinal fluid, Intracranial pressure, Metabolites

Changes in Atrial Natriuretic Polypeptide Receptors in the Choroid Plexus of Experimental Hydrocephalic Rats

Keisuke Tsutsumi,[1] Teruaki Kawano,[1] Kazuo Mori,[1] Masami Niwa,[2] and Masayori Ozaki[1]

[1]Department of Neurosurgery and [2]Department of Pharmacology 2, Nagasaki University School of Medicine, Nagasaki, Japan

We studied the effect of synthetic rat atrial natriuretic polypeptide (1–28) ANF-(99–126) and related atrial natriuretic polypeptides on the accumulation of cyclic GMP (cGMP) in isolated rat choroid plexus in vitro, and changes in choroid plexus ANF-(99–126) bindings in the experimental hydrocephalic rats, the objective being to determine, whether ANF-(99–126) binding sites are physiologically active receptors. One μM of ANF-(99–126) increased the level of cGMP within 30 seconds and the accumulation reached the maximal level 5 minutes after addition of ANF-(99–126) to the incubation media. Increase in the level of cGMP depended on concentration of the peptide, with a range of 100 pM to 10.0 μM. Intracisternal kaolin injection was performed in 1-week-old rats. Half of the group were decapitated after 3 days and the other half after 3 weekes. At both stages after the kaolin injection, the binding amounts of the choroid plexus in the hydrocephalic groups were significantly higher than those of the control groups. Scatchard analysis revealed an increase in the maximal binding capacity (Bmax). These data indicates that binding sites for ANF-(99–126) in the rat choroid plexus may be physiologically active receptors, possibly linked to the production of cerebrospinal fluid, and that the functional change of the choroid plexus in experimental hydrocephalic rats may also be mediated by rANP receptors.

(Annual Report of the Research Committee of "Hydrocephalus," The Ministry of Health and Welfare of Japan, 1986: 41–46, 1987)

Key words: Atrial natriuretic peptied binding sites, Choroid plexus, Cyclic GMP, Experimental hydrocephalus, Quantitative receptor autoradiography

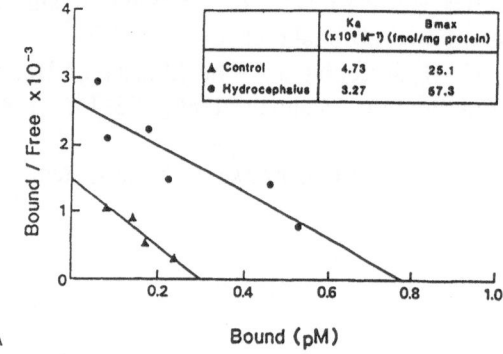

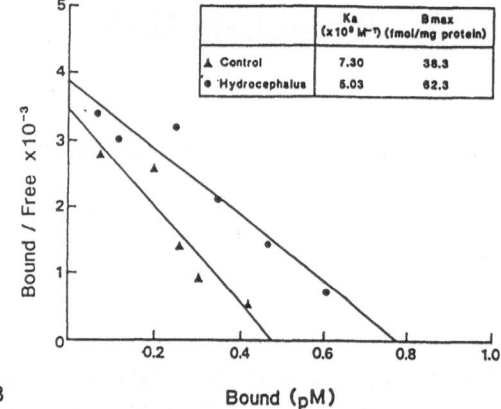

Figure. Scatchard analysis of *I-rANP binding to rat choroid plexus 3 days (**A**) and 3 weeks (**B**) after kaolin injection. ▲: data from control rats. ●: data from hydrocephalic rats. Bmax: binding capacity. Ka: binding affinity.

Changes of Acetylcholinesterase Activity in the Hippocampus of Rats with Kaolin-induced Hydrocephalus: Histochemical study (II)

Masato NAGASAKA, Hiroji KUCHIWAKI, Junki ITOH, Soshun TAKADA, Hitoshi ISHIGURI, and Naoki KAGEYAMA

Department of Neurosurgery, Nagoya University School of Medicine, Nagoya, Japan

It is well known that dementia is one of the major symptoms of the patients with "normal pressure hydrocephalus (NPH)." However, the pathogenesis of the symptom has not fully been understood. Many scientific contributions have appeared on the recently proposed "cholinergic hypothesis of a geriatric memory dysfunction."

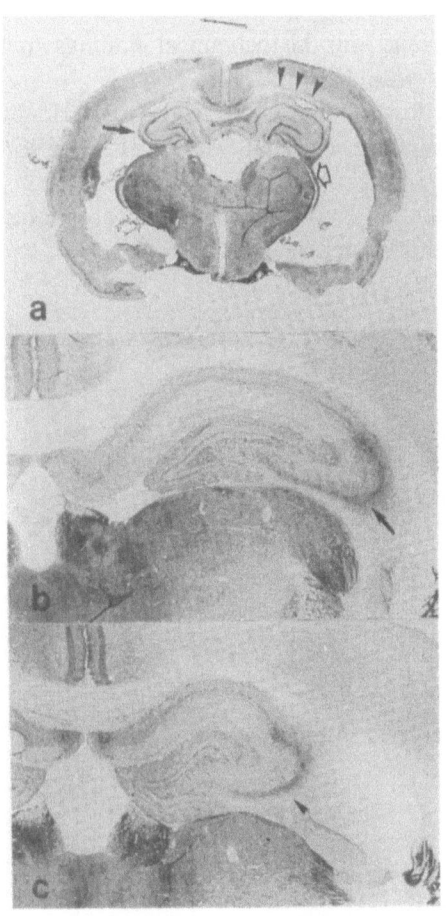

Figure. **a)** Brain slice of hydrocephalic rat in subacute stage shows severe ventriculomegaly, and such histological changes as spongy appearance at the radiatio corporis callosi (*arrowheads*), disruption of the alveus hippocampi (*arrow*) and compression of the fimbria hippocampi (*open arrow*) are noticed (KB staining).
b) Dorsal hippocampus of control rat is shown (AChE staining).
c) Dorsal hippocampus of hydrocephalic rat in chronic stage is shown (AChE staining). At CA3 region (*arrowhead*), activity of AChE decreases in comparison with those of the control rats (b, *arrow*).

The aim of this study is to examine histochemically the effects of hydrocephalus on the acetylcholinesterase (AChE) activity in the hippocampus of adult Wistar rats. An experimental hydrocephalus was produced by the injection of 20% Kaolin suspension into the cisterna magna of the animals. They were grouped into acute, subacute and chronic models according to the conducted time between the injection of Kaolin and the end of the experiment.

At the termination of the experiments, the rats were sacrificed and fixed by cardiac perfusion of 10% buffered formalin. After the degree of the ventriculomegaly was examined, both histochemical staining of AChE (Karnovsky and Roots, 1964) and Klüver-Barrera (KB) staining were performed on the coronal brain slices.

In this study, all the animals which survived the experiments (47%), showed various degrees of hydrocephalus. The rats with severe ventriculomegaly were most frequently observed in subacute stage (*Figure a*), in which most remarkable changes in the white matter were spongy appearances at the radiatio corporis callosi, disruptions of the alveus hippocampi and compressions of the fimbria hippocampi. Additionally, findings of the definitive decrease of AChE activity were noticed around the pyramidal cells of the dorsal hippocampus, especially at the CA3 (Lorente de Nó) region throughout acute and subacute as well as chronic models (*Figure b, c*). The compressed fimbria hippocampi also showed the decrease of AChE activity. These results may demonstrate the impairment of the septo-hippocampal projection in Kaolin-induced hydrocephalic rats.

In conclusion, correlations between hydrocephalus and our histochemical findings may suggest a pathogenesis of the dementia of patients with NPH.

(Annual Report of the Research Committee of "Hydrocephalus," The Ministry of Health and Welfare of Japan, 1986: 31–39, 1987)

Key words: Normal pressure hydrocephalus, Dementia, Kaolin-induced hydrocephalus, Septo-hippocampal projection, Acetylcholinesterase

Changes of Muscarinic Cholinergic Receptors and Cholinergic Neurons in Experimental Hydrocephalus

Koreaki Mori and Takashi Sakamoto

Department of Neurosurgery, Kochi Medical School, Nankoku, Japan

Recently, the relationship between neurological disorders and neurotransmitters has received much attention. Many studies have been reported about the changes of neurotransmitters and their metabolites in cerebrospinal fluid (CSF) in hydrocephalus, and it is presumed that neurotransmitters may play a role in the regulation of CSF dynamics. We injected kaolinum suspension into the cisterna magna of rats and created experimental hydrocephalus. Here we define the acute hydrocephalic stage to be the seventh day after injection and the chronic to be the twenty-first day after injection. We made studies about the changes of muscarinic cholinergic receptors in experimental hydrocephalic rat brains using binding assay, macroautoradiography, and microautoradiography with ^{3}H-quinuclidinyl benzilate (QNB), which has a high and specific affinity for muscarinic receptors. We also studied the changes of cholinergic neurons in experimental hydrocephalic rat brains by immunohistochemical methods with anti-choline acetyltransferase (CAT), the antibody for the synthetic enzyme of acetylcholine which is thought to exist only in cholinergic neurons. Muscarinic cholinergic receptors were increased in acute hydrocephalus, and tended to normalize in chronic hydrocephalus but no change was observed in its distribution. There seemed to be no difference in the number of CAT positive cells between normal and hydrocephalic rat brains, but in hydrocephalic rat brain, CAT positive cells were compressed by the dilated ventricles, and they might have fallen into hypofunction.

It is thought that muscarinic receptors were increased by some mechanism like denervation hypersensitivity because of the reduction of ACh production or release. Recent advancement of PET or SPECT has made it possible to investigate the changes of neurotransmitter receptors in human brain. Such biochemical examination may offer some information to assess the functional state of hydrocephalus and to find a new approach to its treatment. (Annual Report of the Research Committee of "Hydrocephalus," The Ministry of Health and Welfare of Japan, 1986: 23–30, 1987)

Key words: Hydrocephalus, Neurotransmitter, Acetylcholine, Cholinergic neuron, Muscarinic receptor

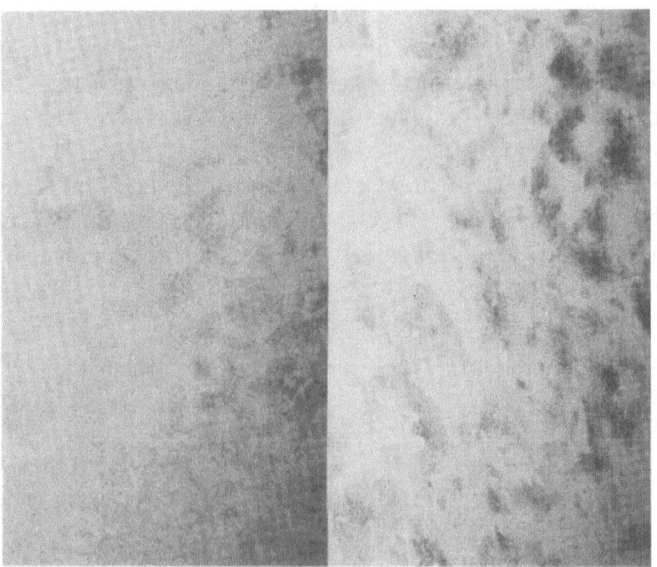

Figure. Microautoradiography of normal rat hippocampus (*left*) and hydrocephalic rat hippocampus (*right*) (×200). The density is higher in hydrocephalic rat hippocampus.

The CSF-level of Uric Acid and γ-aminobutyric Acid in the Hydrocephalus Model of Rabbits

Satoru MOROOKA, Toshinori KANKI, and Norio NAKAMURA

Department of Neurosurgery, Jikei University School of Medicine, Tokyo, Japan

Some cases having the same symptoms as those with normal pressure hydrocephalus (NPH) are unsuccessful in treatment with cerebrospinal fluid (CSF) shunting. Some factors, in combination with the disturbed CSF circulation, derived from the brain tissue are considered to play a role on the onset of NPH. Uric acid and γ-aminobutyric acid (GABA) in CSF were measured in the hydrocephalus models of rabbits. Hydrocephalic state was made by kaolin (Al_2O_3 $2SiO_2$ $2H_2O$) injection. In the fourteen untreated rabbits, the level of uric acid was 62.6 ± 18.3 ng/ml (mean $\pm$ standard deviation) and in the two hydrocephalus models that was elevated from 56.2 to 348 ng/ml and from 89.9 to 247 respectively.

The results were controversial in comparison with measurements in the clinical analysis of NPH in which uric acid level was lower than the control study. It is probable in a human NPH to consider that the turn-over of nucleic acids is supressed which results in low level of uric acid in CSF.

On the other hand, in the experimental hydrocephalus using rabbits, it is rather stressed that destructed cerebral tissue may release uric acid in CSF and results in the elevation of the level of uric acid. In the ten untreated rabbits, the level of GABA was 1.82 ± 1.30 mol/ml. One hydrocephalus model showed the elevated level of GABA from 0.76 to 10.6 nmol/ml. This may indicate the release of GABA in the acute stage of the cerebral ischemia as well as the disturbance of the CSF circulation. This experimental model of the hydrocephalus does not provide with the same pathophysiology of the human NPH, in which loss of functional reserve seems to be characteristic.

(Annual Report of the Research Committee of "Hydrocephalus," The Ministry of Health and Welfare of Japan, 1986: 47–50, 1987)

Key words: Hydrocephalus model, GABA, Uric acid, Kaolin

Table. The levels of GABA and uric acid are elevated in the hydrocephalus models

	BW (kg)	GABA (nmol/ml)	UA (ng/ml)

control rabbit
  mean+standard
    deviation
	3.23±0.43	1.82±1.30	62.6±18.3

experimental rabbit No. 1
  normal state
  hydrocephalic state
	3.3
	2.6
		0.76
		10.6
			56.2
			348

experimental rabbit No. 2
  normal state
  hydrocephalic state
	3.5
	3.0
		
		17.5
			89.9
			247

GABA: γ-aminobutyric acid
UA: Uric acid

The Concentrations of Xanthine and Hypoxanthine in Cerebrospinal Fluid as Therapeutic Guides in Hydrocephalus

Manuel Castro-Gago,[1] Santiago Lojo,[2] Ramón Del Río,[2] Inés Novo,[1] Santiago Rodriguez-Segade,[2] and Antonio Rodríguez[1]

[1]Department of Pediatrics, Neuropediatrics Service; and [2]Central Laboratory Service, Hospital General de Galicia, School of Medicine, University of Santiago de Compostela, Santiago de Compostela, Spain

In treating infantile hydrocephalus it is frequently necessary to decide whether it is better to implant a shunt or to wait for spontaneous improvement. There are presently no universally accepted criteria on which to base this decision. Recently, high levels of oxypurine have been measured in the CSF of hydrocephalic children.

Eighteen hydrocephalic infants ranging from newborn to 4 years of age (mean age=8 months) were monitored throughout 1985. The hydrocephalus was communicating in 9 cases and obstructive in the other 9. Shunts were necessary in all the obstructive cases and in one of the communicating hydrocephalics. No therapeutic action was required in the 8 communicating hydrocephalus patients with Evans indexes between 0.32 and 0.41, whose psychomotor development over the 12 months was considered normal, with no increase in ventricular size as measured by real time ultrasound and by computerized tomography. They were, accordingly, seemed to have self-compensated. The xanthine, hypoxanthine and total oxypurine levels in the CSF of all hydrocephalic patients and 8 healthy controls to obtain the normal range (non-hydrocephalic emergency patients with normal CSF) were measured by HPLC. Levels were determined again in all the children who required a shunt 15 days after its implantation. The results were analyzed statistically, using de Student's t-test.

The mean xanthine, hypoxanthine and total oxypurine levels in the normal children were 5.20, 5.59 and 11.29 nmol/l, respectively. In self-compensated hydrocephalics these levels were respectively 6.06, 6.50 and 12.57 nmol/l. In non-compensated hydrocephalics, they were 11.40, 10.79 and 22.19 nmol/l. The differences between the latter group and the first two are statistically significant ($p < 0.001$) (*Table*). Fifteen days after implantation of shunts in the non-compensated hydrocephalics, the mean xanthine levels had fallen to 4.61 nmol/l, the mean hypoxanthine levels to 5.03 nmol/l, and the mean total oxypurine levels to 9.64 nmol/l. The change is statistically significant ($p < 0.001$).

In light of these findings we propose that xanthine, hypoxanthine and total oxypurine levels be used in cases of hydrocephalus as guides for therapeutic action and to monitor progress.

(Child's Nerv Syst 2: 109–111, 1986)

Key words: Hydrocephalus, Cerebrospinal fluid, Total oxypurines, Xanthine, Hypoxanthine

	X̄±SD		
	Hypoxanthine	Xanthine	Total oxypurine
Controls (8)	5.94±0.74	5.20±0.87	11.29±1.11
Self-compensated (8)	6.50±0.86	6.06±1.62	12.57±2.30
Non-compensated (10)	10.68±1.55	11.40±1.54	22.19±2.89

Table.

Hypoxanthine, xanthine and total oxypurine in the CSF of patients and controls. The differences between the hypoxanthine, xanthine, and total oxypurine levels of the non-compensated patients and those of the other two groups are statistically significant ($p<0.001$).

Immune Complex Assay in Infantile Hydrocephalus

Adebayo KAZEEM

Department of Clinical Pathology, School of Clinical Sciences, College of Medicine, University of Lagos, Lagos, Nigeria

The acceptable treatment modality for the abnormal accummulation of cerebrospinal fluid as hydrocephalus is shunt procedure, and this surgical device can become complicated by infection with the possible breakdown of the blood-brain-barrier (BBB). With this background concept, we used laser immunonephelometry to quantitate and compare the immune complexes in the hydrocephalic fluid (HCF) and their serum, using the lumbar cerebrospinal fluid (CSF) of non-hydrocephalic fluid infants as control.

Our results revealed that the values of IgG, IgA and IgM complexes in the HCF were relatively low compared to those of their serum. The value of IgM complex in the HCF was so very low that this could not be computed from our IgM standard curve. These observations were interpreted as follows:

(i)   There was no evidence of selective admixture of immune complexes between the blood vascular compartment and the HCF space,

(ii)   The lack of selective increase of immune complexes in the HCF comparable to that of the blood suggested that the BBB may be intact in infantile hydrocephalus.

When the values of immune complexes in the HCF were compared with those of the lumbar CSF of non-hydrocephalic infants the only observation was the IgG gradient. The limited scope of our study could not provide an explanation backed by scientific data but we thought the IgG gradient was probably related to flow dynamics rather than de-novo synthesis. In general, the low levels of the immune complexes in the HCF when associated with artificial shunt device implantation for the treatment of the hydrocephalus may be a predisposing factor that can lead to overwhelming infection among this group of patients.

(Child's Nerv Syst 2: 252–254, 1986)

Key words: Immune complexes, Hydrocephalus, Infantile shunt procedure

Table.

Class of Immune Complexes	Values (mg/d*l*)*		
	Hydrocephalic Infants		Non-hydrocephalic Infants
	Serum	Hydrocephalic fluid	Lumbar C & F
IgG	2283±13.26	2810.9± 4.8	2440.8±2.0
IgA	212±65.4	26.4±14.5	28.6±1.8
IgM	320±59.4	below estimation	

*Value=Mean±SD

II) Pathophysiology

Hydrodynamics
Intracranial Pressure
Etiopathogenesis

CSF Dynamics in Children:
A quantitative analysis of the relativity of major and minor pathways of cerebro-spinal fluid dynamics

Shizuo Oi,[1] Yoshiteru Shose,[1] Hiroshi Yamada,[2] Akihiro Ijichi,[2] and Satoshi Matsumoto[2]

Department of Neurosurgery, [1]National Kagawa Children's Hospital, Zentsuji; and [2]Kobe University, Kobe, Japan

Cerebrospinal fluid (CSF) dynamics in infants and children is still obscure. This paper aims to analyze the characteristics of CSF dynamics in the younger age group and to clarify the changes both in the acute/chronic hydrocephalic status and in the post-shunt condition on the basis of our experience with 118 cases of metrizamide CT cisternography. In order to pursue the CSF passive movements, the exact regional CT numbers were obtained by means of the ROI method in each case at 3, 6, and 24 hours after metrizamide injection.

The results revealed that, in the normal CSF dynamics in both the major and minor pathways in children, it took more than 24 hours until the regional metrizamide was completely cleared up.

In the acute hydrocephalic state, the ventricular reflux and stasis of the contrast was remarkable, and stagnation in the Sylvian fissure continued more than 24 hours. In the minor pathway, the contrast moved into the brain parenchyma, with there obviously being more in the subependymal layer and the adjacent white matter, and lasted more than 24 hours. On the other hand, these phenomena were very much less prominent in the chronic phase of hydrocephalus. This fact may suggest the hypothesis that a reconstituted active major or minor fluid pathway does not play an important role in the compensation of the acute high-pressure progressive hydrocephalic state.

The CSF dynamics in a shunted hydrocephalus are obviously improved when in stasis or when stagnated inside or outside of the ventricular system. The timing of the metrizamide clear-up was within 24 hours after achieving a high accumulation of the contrast in the lateral ventricle where the shunt is placed. The contrast movement in the brain parenchyma as the minor pathway was significantly less in a shunted hydrocephalus, and there was almost none in cases of slit-like ventricles.   (*CT Kenkyu* 8 (2): 153–162, 1986)

Key words: CSF dynamics, Infants and children, Acute hydrocephalus, Compensated hydrocephalus, Slit-like ventricle

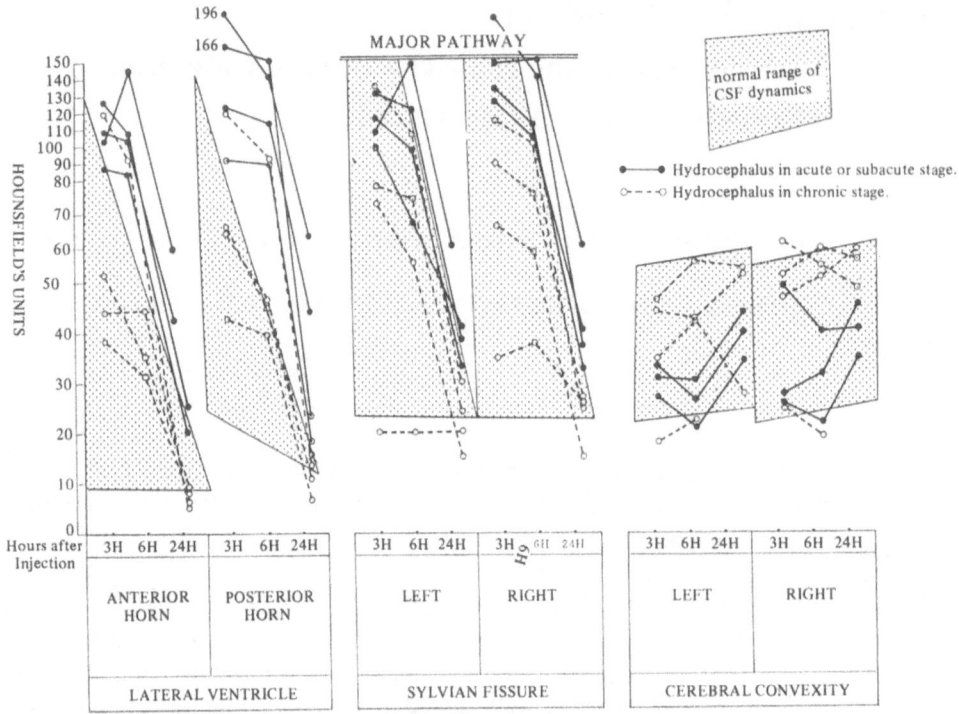

Figure 1. CSF dynamics in major pathway in acute/chronic hydrocephalic state in children.

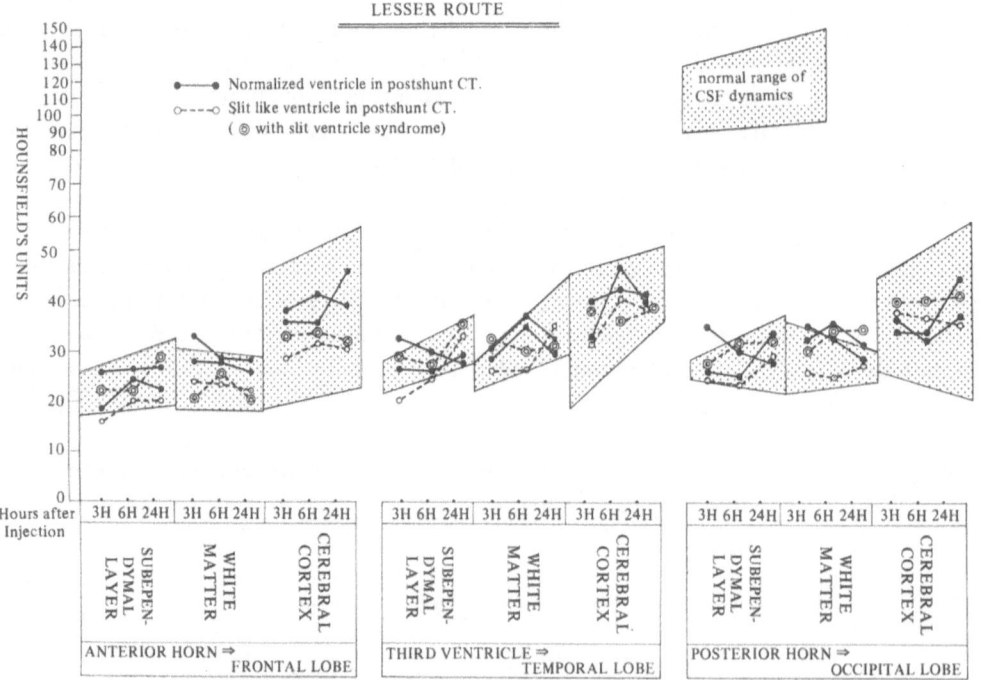

Figure 2. CSF dynamics in minor pathway in postshunt hydrocephalic state in children.

The Value of CSF Flow Studies in Infants with Communicating Hydrocephalus

Francesco Velardi,[1] Harold J. Hoffman,[2] Judith M. Ash,[3] E. Bruce Hendrick,[2] and Robin P. Humphreys[2]

[1]Division of Neurosurgery, Università Cattolica del S. Cuore, L. go Gemelli Rome, Italy; [2]Division of Neurosurgery and [3]Division of Nuclear Medicine, University of Toronto and the Hospital for Sick Children, Toronto, Ontario, Canada

Infants presenting with macrocephaly are often encountered in a pediatric clinical practice leaving the clinician often uncertain when faced with borderline dilatation of cerebrospinal fluid (CSF) spaces or, even more, when the CT scan shows an accumulation of fluid over the convexities, with relative preservation of normal ventricular size. In such situations, the dynamic detection of CSF pathways can provide helpful answers as to whether a shunting procedure is necessary. The uselfuness of isotopic CSF scanning in investigating such patients is described in this study.

Results of the scan were analyzed by an experienced observer and designated according to their features, into 1 of 4 arbitrarily defined groups (*Table 1*).

Results of the isotopic CSF scanning and need for shunting are summarized in *Table 2*. *DISCUSSION*: in infants under 1 year of age, the combination of enlarged CSF spaces and macrocephaly is not always a manifestation of progressive hydrocephalus. The ability to predict the evolution of patients with increased head growth rate and abnormal CT findings is particularly important at this age in order to avoid macrocephaly and permanent neurological impairment.

In our experience, CSF scanning and the grading scheme we used to score its features has proved to be a reliable indicator of the presence and degree of CSF flow impairment. None of the patients with grade I CSF scan needed a shunt procedure, while all patients but one with grades III and IV showed rapid progression of the disease, leading to surgical treatment of the underlying hydrocephalus. Only 7 of 18 patients with a grade II CSF flow disturbance eventually needed a surgical procedure. This was due to the progression of clinical signs over a short period of observation, during which some of the patients underwent direct ICP monitoring. Moreover, the demonstration of spatial continuity of the presumed effusion with the subarachnoid space, as witnessed by its filling with radioactive tracer through a

Table 1. Grading of CSF flow study

Grade	Ventricular filling	Flow over the convexities
I	No	Yes
II	Yes; out by 24 h	Yes
III	Yes; persistent at 24 h	Yes
IV	Yes; persistent at 24 h	No

Table 2. Grading of disordered CSF dynamic in relation to mode of management

Grade of CSF scan	Number of patients	Surgical treatment required	
		Yes	No
I	6	—	6
II	18	7	11
III	8	7	1
IV	2	2	—

subarachnoid lumbar injection, is helpful in the differential diagnosis. It also supports the treatment by means of a lumboperitoneal shunt because it confirms the communicating nature of the hydrocephalus.   (Child's Nerv Syst 2: 139–143, 1986)

Key words: CSF scan, Hydrocephalus, Intraventricular hemorrhage, Macrocephaly, Prematurity

The CSF Pulse Wave in Hydrocephalus

Harold D. PORTNOY

Oakland Neurological Clinic, P.C., Bloomfield Hills, MI, USA

This was a letter to the editor in response to comments by C. Di Rocco criticizing the paper "The CSF pulse wave in hydrocephalus" (Child's Nerv Syst 1:248–254). Di Rocco did not agree with our comment that the CSF pressure pulse emanates from the cerebral venous bed but rather is "significant only in conditions of increased return of venous blood to the heart." Our studies indicate that 1) the pulse is not transmitted from the heart in a retrograde manner because obstruction of the transverse sinuses in dogs with diversion of the venous outflow failed to obliterate the sagittal sinus pulse. 2) the pulse wave measured in the CSF and in the cerebral veins are identical. Thus, the pulse originates in the veins and is transmitted to the CSF, or vice versa. If the pulse originates in the CSF, it must come from some vascular structure in contact with the CSF. The usual explanation is that the pulse originates in the arteries at the base of the brain and is modified by 'compliance' of the system with the pulse impressed upon the cerebral veins acting as a tambour. CSF and venous pulse waves were measured in our laboratory so as to eliminate the tambour effect. The pulse waves were still identical. We are left with the conclusion that the venous pulse is an antegrade phenomena and is transmitted from the veins to the CSF. As regards asymmetric ventricles in a shunted patient, the pressure gradient is not between the ventricles. The gradient is between the intracranial contents and the distal end of the shunt. This causes CSF and the viscoelastic brain to flow toward the ventricular catheter. The tendency to flow is more dispersed the further the ventricular surface is from the pressure sink, *i.e.,* the ventricular catheter. Thus the ventricle with the catheter is the smaller ventricle.

(Child's Nerv Syst 2: 107–108, 1986)

Key words: CSF pulse wave, Venous pulse, Ventriculomegaly

Analysis of CSF Dynamics by Computerized Pressure-elastance Resorption Test in Hydrocephalic Children: Indications for surgery

J. Woojan, M. Roszkowski, S. Sliwka, L. Batorski, and G. Pawlowski

Department of Pediatric Neurosurgery, Children's Memorial Hospital, Child Health Center, Warsaw, Poland

Hydrocephalus and its optimal treatment present the clinician with one of the most difficult problems in childhood diseases. Progress in diagnostic possibilities in recent years, has permitted better understanding of the pathomechanisms of this affection; a spinal steady-state infusion test may be considered as one of the best methods for studying intracranial hydrodynamics. The infusion curves obtained were processed by a specialized computer system to obtain principal parameters describing the CSF dynamics for each patient. The calculations were based on our mathematical model of cerebrospinal fluid compensatory mechanisms. Since 1982, 23 hydrocephalic children have been studied. Computerized analysis of the P/V and AMP/P curves provides valuable data that describe precisely the degree of disturbances of CSF dynamics. The following parameters were quantitatively determined: outflow resistance (R), resting pressure (P1), elastance (e), elastivity (alfa), reference pressure (P$\emptyset$) and optimum (break-point) pressure (Popt).

On the basis of our observations we were able to divide our patients into four groups according to the parameters of intracranial compensation (*Table*). In the first group, the results of the infusion test were normal. These children were then followed up as outpatients, studied with CT and psychologic tests. In the second, third, and fourth groups, increased outflow resistance was observed. In the second group, the intracranial pressure compensated at a higher level (chronic hydrocephalus); in the third group the outflow resistance, resting pressure, elastance and elastivity were elevated, but the intracranial pressure was not compensated (acute hydrocephalus); in the fourth group, cases of Dandy-Walker syndrome, there was also noted an elevated value of PO, probably a result of impaired venous outflow.

In the last three groups, operative treatment consisted of either a ventriculoatrial, ventriculoperitoneal, or a lumboperitoneal shunt.

It is concluded that the described test allows the differential diagnosis of hydrocephalus in children.   (Child's Nerv Syst 2: 98–100, 1986)

Key words: Hydrocephalus, CSF dynamics, Elastance

Table. Four clinical groups divided up according to the parameters of intracranial space (N-normal, I-increased, D-decreased)

Type of hydro-cephalus	Results of infusion test					Conclusions
	R	Pl	e	Pø	Popt	
Ex vacuo	N	N	N/D	N	N	Brain atrophy Shunt ineffective
Chronic	I	N/I	N/D	N	I	Shunt indicated
Acute	I	I	I	N	N	Shunt necessary
Dandy-Walker syndrome	N/I	I	N/I	I	I	Shunt necessary

Variations in Pressure-volume Index and CSF Outflow Resistance at Different Locations in the Feline Craniospinal Axis

Hideo Takizawa, Thea Gabra-Sanders, and J. Douglas Miller

Department of Surgical Neurology, University of Edinburgh, Edinburgh, Scotland

Pressure volume index (PVI) and cerebrospinal fluid (CSF) outflow resistance (R_0) were estimated in spontaneously breathing anesthetized cats by the bolus injection test under normal conditions and also under abnormal conditions produced by slow infusion of saline into the CSF space. Bolus injections were made separately into the lumbar subarachnoid space, cisterna magna, and lateral ventricle. The mean PVI values in the lumbar sac, cisterna magna, and lateral ventricle under normal conditions were 0.70, 0.71, and 0.64 m*l*, respectively; not significantly different from each other. Saline infusion lowered PVI significantly at every site; PVI values in the lumbar sac, cisterna magna, and lateral ventricle were 0.54, 0.52, and 0.53 m*l*, respectively; not significantly different from each other. Indirect values of PVI were calculated from the pressure responses observed at sites other than where the bolus had been injected. These indirect PVI values were always greater than PVI at the injection site under normal conditions, but differences between direct and indirect PVI values were abolished during saline loading of the CSF space. The R_0 was estimated under normal conditions in the lumbar sac, cisterna magna, and lateral ventricle to be 81.6, 85.6, and 110.3 mm Hg/ml/min, respectively. The lateral ventricle R_0 was significantly higher than at other places. These findings suggest that, when there is no blockage in the craniospinal axis, the pressure response to a bolus change in CSF volume is freely transmitted, direct measurements of PVI are independent of location, and indirect measurements are larger because of "buffering" in the CSF space. When PVI is lowered and buffering capacity is exhausted, these differences between direct and indirect PVI values disappear. (J Neurosurg 64: 298–303, 1986)

Key words: Intracranial pressure, Pressure-volume index, Cerebrospinal fluid outflow, Resistance, Cat

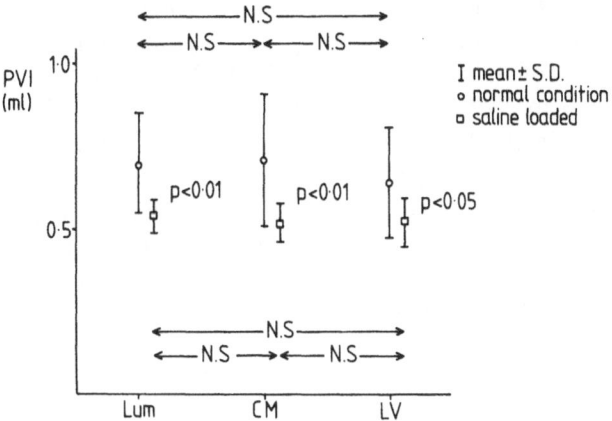

Figure. Variations of direct pressure-volume index (PVI) values in the lumbar sac (Lum), cisterna magna (CM), and lateral ventricle (LV) under normal conditions (*circles*) and saline loading (*squares*). Mean values±standard deviations (S.D.) are shown. NS=not significant.

CSF Dynamics and Pressure-volume Relationships in Communicating Hydrocephalus

Michael Kosteljanetz

Department of Neurosurgery, Aalborg Sygehus, Aalborg, Denmark

Normal-pressure hydrocephalus or communicating hydrocephalus are more or less synonymous designations of a potentially treatable condition. Twenty-nine patients with this diagnosis were studied. In 17 cases the etiology was unknown. In 3 patients etiology was subarachnoid hemorrhage. The following studies were undertaken. 1) continuous intracranial pressure (ICP) monitoring by means of an intraventricular catheter; 2) pressure-volume studies; and 3) measurement of resistance to outflow of cerebrospinal fluid (R_{out}). The two latter were studied by the bolus injection or pressure-volume index (PVI) technique. In 19 patients mean ICP never exceeded 15 mmHg. In the other 10 patients varying degrees of mildly raised ICP was noted. The frequency of 1/2 to 2/min. waves varied from 3% to 58%. PVI ranged from 4.6 to 18.2 ml, which is below what is considered normal limits. No explanation for this highly abnormal pressure-volume condition could be offered.

The R_{out} ranged from 2.5 to 31.4 mmHg and was linearly correlated to the ICP (correlation coefficient=0.80). Thus, patients with a higher R_{out} also had a higher ICP as compared with patients with lower R_{out}, yet ICP could still be within limits considered normal. Cerebrospinal fluid dynamics (formation rate x resistance) contributed much more to the ICP than in normal individuals (where it is estimated to contribute approximately 10%). It is postulated that communicating hydrocephalus represents one endpoint of a continuum, where the preceeding phase is high-pressure and high-resistance hydrocephalus as for

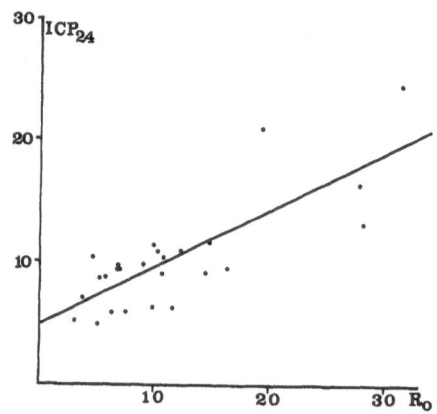

Figure. Plot of resistance to cerebrospinal fluid outflow (R_o in mmHg/ml/min.) versus the average overnight (24 hours) intracranial pressure (ICP_{24} in mmHg). The linear regression line is shown.

instance, is seen after subarachnoid hemorrhage and after experimental hydrocephalus. In some patients there is a possibility of cerebral atrophy accompanied by otherwise insignificant increased R_{out}. In this study the PVI technique proved to be a fast and safe method of measuring R_{out}. However, there was no prove with regard to the predictive value of R_{out} measurements in the selection of patients for CSF-shunting.

(J Neurosurg 64: 45–52, 1986)

Key words: Communicating hydrocephalus, Normal-pressure hydrocephalus, Intracranial pressure, Pressure-volume index, Cerebrospinal fluid dynamics

Cerebrospinal Fluid Pulse Pressure and the Pulsatile Variation in Cerebral Blood Volume:
An experimental study in dogs

John H. M. van Eijndhoven and Cees J. J. Avezaat

Central Department of Automation Informatics (CDAI) and Department of Neurosurgery, Academic Hospital Rotterdam-Dijkzigt, Rotterdam, The Netherlands

The cerebrospinal fluid pulse pressure (CSFPP) has found application as a measure of intracranial elastance. However, CSFPP is also dependent on the magnitude of the pulsatile variation in cerebral blood volume (ΔV_b). The purpose of the present study was to assess the effect on ΔV_b of changes in systemic arterial pressure (SAP) and arterial carbon dioxide tension ($PaCO_2$) as well as elevation of intracranial pressure (ICP). Therefore, ΔV_b was computed from the electromagnetically measured flow profile in the vertebral artery of the dog on the assumption of a nonpulsatile cerebral venous outflow (see *figure*).

During arterial hypotension, ΔV_b was increased due to a shift of flow from diastole to systole, whereas mean flow was not affected. The reverse phenomenon was observed when SAP was raised. Changes in $PaCO_2$ had little effect on pulsatile blood flow. The changes in total blood flow that occurred were evenly distributed over the cardiac cycle. Consequently, ΔV_b was not significantly affected, although CSFPP was considerably changed. When ICP was raised, a breakpoint pressure was observed above which cerebral blood flow (CBF) decreased and CSFPP and ΔV_b increased. This contradiction was explained by the finding of a decrease in diastolic flow, causing the fall in CBF, whereas systolic flow relative to mean flow was increased, resulting in an increased ΔV_b. The underlying mechanisms of the pulsatile flow changes are extensively discussed. It is argued that the arterial inflow profile is largely determined by the compliance of the inflow section of the cerebral vascular bed. Vascular compliance is significantly altered by changes in SAP and ICP because they affect the transmural pressure of the vessels, whereas this is not the case during changes in $PaCO_2$.

(Neurosurgery 19: 507–522, 1986)

Key words: Cerebral blood volume, Cerebrospinal fluid pulse pressure, Electromagnetic flowmetry, Intracranial elastance, Intracranial pressure

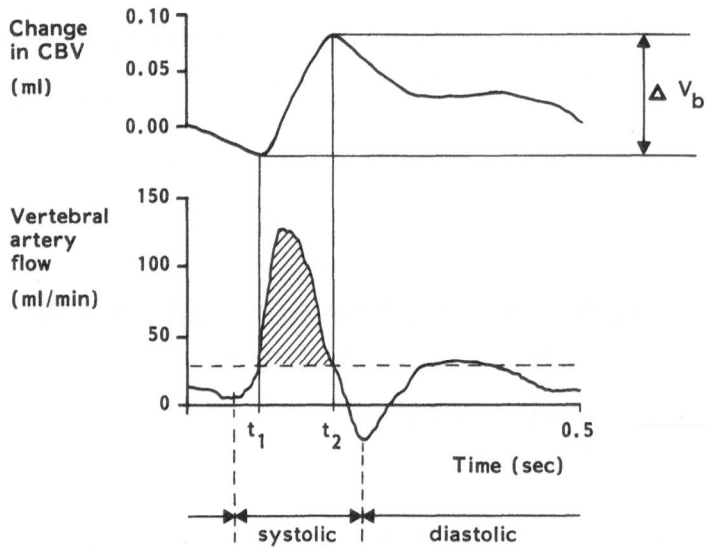

Figure. Vertebral artery blood flow and computed change in CBV during one cardiac cycle in an experimental animal. Mean flow level, which is equal to venous outflow if this is assumed to be nonpulsatile, is given by dashed line. During time interval t_1-t_2, inflow of cerebral blood exceeds outflow, causing an increase in CBV. Magnitude of pulsatile change in CBV (ΔV_b) is determined by difference between extreme values of CBV.

Relationship Between Respiration and Pressure Wave:
An experimental study in kaolin-induced hydrocephalus

Yukihiko UEDA, Takashi MATSUMOTO, Mitsuhito MASE, and Hajime NAGAI

Department of Neurosurgery, Nagoya City University Medical School, Nagoya, Japan

Plateau waves often are observed in patients with "normal pressure hydrocephalus" during continuous monitoring of intracranial pressure (ICP). An experiment was performed to determine whether respiratory changes cause plateau waves in patients with hydrocephalus

Table. Changes in blood gas, heart rate (HR), systemic arterial pressure (SAP), ICP and CPP caused by hypoventilation (1) and difference of response to hypoventilation among groups (2)

1.

		Normoventi. state (N) (Mean±S.D.)	Hypoventi. state (H) (Mean±S.D.)	Statistical significance between N and H (t-test)
Control group (C) <4 cases>	pH	7.36± 0.03	7.12± 0.09	P<0.01
	PaCO$_2$ (mmHg)	36.7 ± 2.9	73.2 ±15.6	P<0.02
	HR (/min.)	156.5 ±33.3	105.8 ±25.6	P<0.05
	mean SAP (mmHg)	139.5 ±14.6	163.5 ±22.6	P<0.05
	mean ICP (mmHg)	6.0 ± 2.8	36.0 ± 6.5	P<0.01
	CPP (mmHg)	133.5 ±14.1	127.5 ±16.1	N.S.
Kaolin Hyd. group (K) <4 cases>	pH	7.38± 0.02	7.19± 0.04	P<0.01
	PaCO$_2$ (mmHg)	33.3 ± 2.0	56.0 ± 6.3	P<0.01
	HR (/min.)	160.0 ±13.8	96.3 ±20.8	P<0.05
	mean SAP (mmHg)	157.7 ±60.1	167.3 ±44.5	N.S.
	mean ICP (mmHg)	11.2 ± 4.5	64.2 ±22.4	P<0.05
	CPP (mmHg)	146.4 ±63.5	103.1 ±53.7	N.S.
Ballon group (B) <4 cases>	pH	7.36± 0.03	7.15± 0.08	P<0.01
	PaCO$_2$ (mmHg)	38.0 ± 3.2	68.4 ± 8.7	P<0.01
	HR (/min.)	135.5 ±30.9	116.8 ±34.9	N.S.
	mean SAP (mmHg)	126.0 ±31.7	144.0 ±21.3	N.S.
	mean ICP (mmHg)	12.2 ± 1.9	60.7 ± 7.7	P<0.01
	CPP (mmHg)	113.8 ±29.9	83.3 ±15.5	P<0.1

2.

	Control group (C) <4 cases> (Mean±S.D.)	Kaolin Hyd. group (K) <4 cases> (Mean±S.D.)	Ballon group (B) <4 cases> (Mean±S.D.)	Statistical significance between C and K (t-test)	Statistical significance between C and B (t-test)	Statistical significance between K and B (t-test)
mean SAP (mmHg)	163.5±22.6	167.3±44.5	144.0±21.3	N.S.	N.S.	N.S.
mean ICP (mmHg)	36.0± 6.5	64.2±22.4	60.7± 7.7	P<0.1	P<0.01	N.S.
CPP (mmHg)	127.5±16.1	103.5±53.7	83.3±15.5	N.S.	P<0.02	N.S.

and normal ICP. Twelve adult mongrel dogs were immobilized and ventilated mechanically. Hypoventilation for ten minutes was induced by decreasing both the tidal volume and the respiratory rate to half those of normal ventilation, and then normal ventilation was resumed. The dogs were divided into three groups; Control group, 4 dogs (Group C); Kaolin-induced hydrocephalus group, in which the ICP had returned to the normal range in chronic stage, 4 dogs (Group K); and, for the purpose of comparison to Group K, an extradural balloon-inflated group in which the ICP was within the normal range, 4 dogs (Group B). During hypoventilation, the level of increased ICP was higher, and in response to changes in ICP, cerebral perfusion pressure (CPP) was decreased significantly more in Group

K and Group B than in Group C. The increase in ICP persisted during hypoventilation, as do plateau waves. None of the parameters monitored showed any statistically significant difference between Group K and Group B, therefore the response of ICP in these two groups probably is similar for the same respiratory changes.

These results suggest that the spatial compensatory capacity of kaolin-induced hydrocephalus is decreased even if the ICP is within the normal range. In such physical circumstances, changes in the cerebral blood volume caused by respiratory changes can induce inceased ICP which persists as plateau waves. It also is suggested that changes in respiration might be one of the factors that causes plateau waves in normal pressure hydrocephalus in man.

(Annual Report of the Research Committee of "Hydrocephalus," The Ministry of Health and Welfare of Japan, 1986: 79–87, 1987)

Key words: Plateau wave, Respiration, Kaolin-induced hydrocephalus, Normal pressure hydrocephalus, Intracranial pressure

Biomechanics of Hydrocephalus:
Part I. Mechanical properties of the brain

Tatsuya Nagashima,[1] Norihiko Tamaki,[1] Satoshi Matsumoto,[1] Tetsuya Tateishi,[2] and Yoshio Shirasaki[2]

[1]Department of Neurosurgery, Kobe University School of Medicine, Kobe; and [2]Department of Biomechanics, Machine Engineering Laboratory, Ibaraki, Japan

In considering the pathophysiology of hydrocephalus in children, it is necessary to consider properties of brain tissue itself in addition to circulation of cerebrospinal fluid. The first step of biomechanical approach to hydrocephalus is to clarify the mechanical properties of brain tissue.

In this paper, mechanical properties of brain tissue were measured by using a biomechanical spectrometer (Rheovibron, Toyo Bowldwin Model DDV-VMF). And micro-wave absorption method was evaluated as a method for measuring *in vivo* mechanical properties of brain tissue. Thirteen rats were used for the *in vivo* experiment. They were devided into 6 groups, control, dead, varying blood pressure, venous ligation, and brain edema group. An burr hole of 10 mm diameter was made at parietal region and creep tests were done with a indenter of 4 mm diameter. In the dead group, the displacement increased 1.2 times of that of the control group and $T_{1/2}$ was shortened from 25 seconds of the control to 12 seconds. In the venous ligation group, the displacement was decreased 0.57 times of that of the control and $T_{1/2}$ shortened from 15 seconds of control to 10.6 seconds. When the blood pressure was changed by the intravenous injection of Angiotensin and exsanguination, the displacement followed the change of the blood pressure. In the brain edema group, the characteristics of micro-wave absorption varied to low frequency side and almost coinsided with that of saline. However, there was no change of return loss.

The results showed that the cerebral arterio-venous system plays an important roles in the mechanical properties of brain tissue. The characteristics of micro-wave absorption represented the change of mechanical properties of brain tissue very well. Therefore, the method is a hopefull clinical method to evaluate *in vivo* mechanical properties of brain tissue. In future, it is necessary to conduct quantitative measurement of the mechanical properties of brain. For this purpose, it is important to make new comprehensive mechanical model which includes brain tissue, cerebrospinal fluid and arteriovenous system. Furthermore it is necessary to develop a new method to analyze the experiments which have material heterogeneity, complex geometry and boundary conditions.

(*Shoni no Noshinkei* 11: 233–238, 1986)

Key words: Hydrocephalus, Biomechanics, Brain, Cerebrospinal fluid

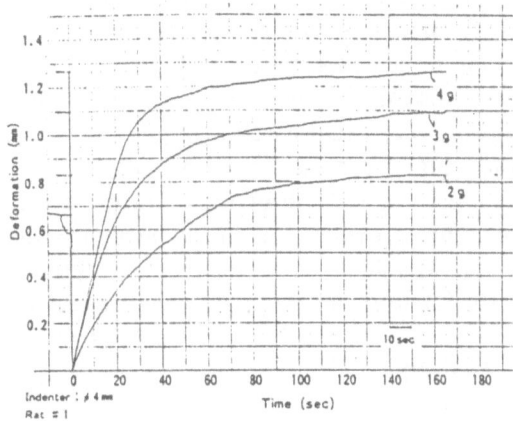

Figure 1. The creep curves which were obtained by constant loading of 2, 3, and 4 gram to the brain surface of normal rat.

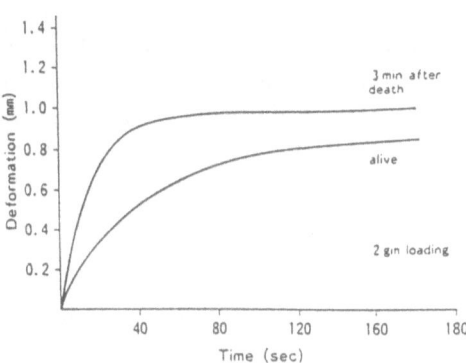

Figure 2. The change of creep curve after death. Two gram of constant loading was applied to the brain surface before and after death.

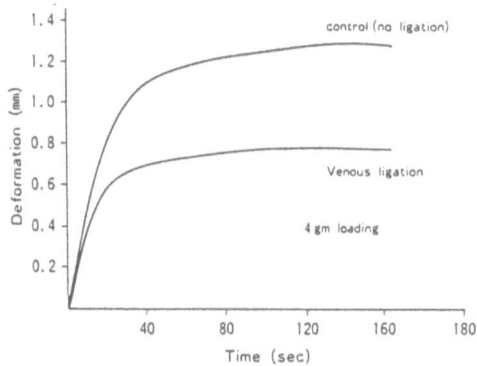

Figure 3. The change of creep curve after ligation of cervical veins.

Fetal Heart Rate Pattern During Decompression of a Hydrocephalic Head: Case report

Miriam Katz, Israel Meizner, Arnon Wiznitzer, and Zion J. Hagay

Department of Obstetrics and Gynecology, Soroka University Hospital; and Faculty of Health Sciences, Ben-Gurion University of the Negev, Beer-Sheva, Israel

A primiparous fundal patient at 40 weeks' gestation was admitted in active labor. The height was 43 cm. Ultrasonic scan demonstrated a hydrocephalic fetal head with B.P.D. of 11.4 cm, and brain thickness of 0.6 cm. Fetal heart rate monitoring revealed severe baseline bradycardia with normal variability and acceleration. To enable vaginal delivery, transabdominal puncture was performed and 400 ml of C. S. F. was drained. During the decompression baseline fetal heart rate changed from severe to moderate bradycardia (*Figure*).
The normal fetal heart rate pattern is the result of interaction between the sympathetic and parasympathetic components of the autonomic nervous system. Elevated intracranial pressure (head compression) has been found to cause persistent baseline bradycardia. It is, therefore, consistent that elevated intracranial pressure caused severe baseline bradycardia in the present case. The drainage of cerebrospinal fluid caused a dramatic shift from overtly abnormal to normal fetal heart rate pattern. This provides convincing evidence that intracranial pressure plays a critical role in the pathophysiology of fetal heart rate patterns.

(Br J Obstet Gynaecol 93: 881–882, 1986)

Key words: Hydrocephalus, Fetal heart rate, Decompression

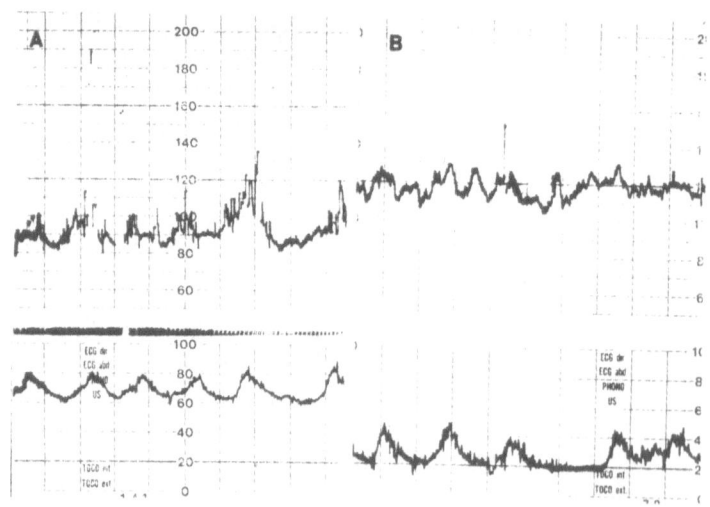

Figure.

X-Linked Hydrocephalus

Ruben I. KUZNIECKY, Gordon V. WATTERS, Lise WATTERS, and Kathleen MEAGHER-VILLEMURE

Departments of Neurology and Pathology, Montreal Children's Hospital, McGill University, Montreal, Canada

Two French-Canadian families with seven cases of hydrocephalus in two generations are presented. The pattern of inheritance is consistent with an X-linked recessive transmission. The clinical and pathologic characteristics of this entity are reviewed. The anomaly of adducted thumbs was present in one patient and its cause is considered. The hypothesis of primary hydrocephalus and secondary compression of the aqueduct as the mechanism for aqueductal stenosis is discussed.   (Can J Neurol Sci 13: 344-346, 1986)

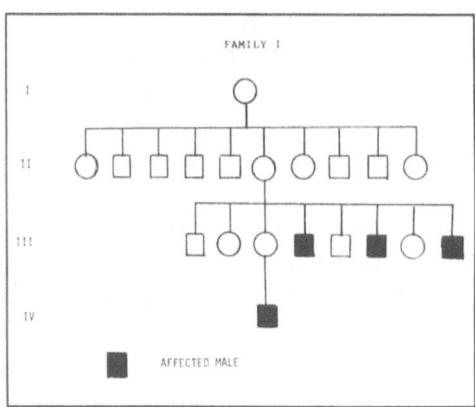

Figure 1. Pedigree of Family I. Patient IV1 is presently alive.

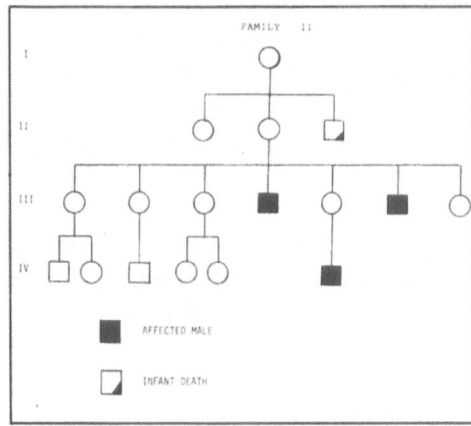

Figure 2. Pedigree of Family II.

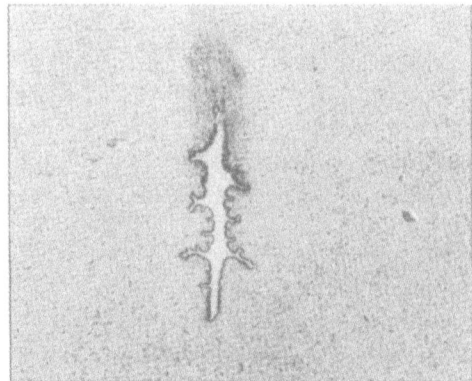

Figure 3. Section through the inferior portion of the Aqueduct, showing stenosis with a normal ependymal lining. (magnification ×50)

A Family of Hereditary Communicating Hydrocephalus

Koh-ichi Mizoguchi and Yoshiro Nishimura

First Department of Internal Medicine, Hamamatsu University School of Medicine, Hamamatsu; Department of Neurology, Shizuoka National Hospital, Shizuoka, Japan

We studied a family of hereditary communicating hydrocephalus with trigonocephaly, affecting four males and four females across three generations. The proband was 51 years old man. Their common clinical features were spastic gait after the third decade and dementia after the fifth decade. On the skull X-ray films, the temporal buldging with thinning of the calvalium and the erosion of the dorsum sellae were demonstrated. CT scans of affected persons showed marked dilatation of ventricles and mild widening of cortical sulci. On R. I. cisternography, performed on four members, the marked dilatation of ventricles and the ventricular reflux during 3 to 72 hours were observed. The radioisotopes were not accumulated in the parasagittal regions through the examination. The findings suggesting the ventricular dilatation and the tourtuous cortical veins close to the superior sagittal sinus were observed on the carotid angiography, performed on three. Their hydrocephalus might be accounted for by the disturbance of the cerebrospinal fluid absorption in the sagittal regions, related to the tourtuous cortical veins.

Many hydrocephalic cases craniosynostosis have been reported previously. They were accompanied by other deformities in either the body or the skull. The hydrocephalus was considered to be induced by the disturbance of the cerebrospinal fluid path due to the severely deformed skull. As the dural sinuses and the cortical veins developed with close

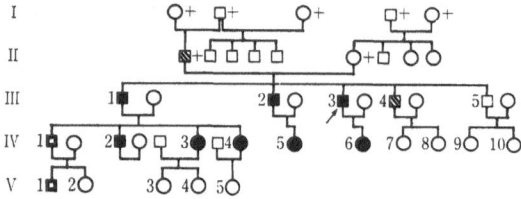

	III-1	III-2	III-3	IV-2	IV-3	IV-4	IV-5	IV-6
Age	61	55	54	35	33	31	23	27
Sex	M	M	M	M	F	F	F	F
Headache	+	−	−	−	−	−	−	−
Memory disturbance	+	+	+	−	−	−	−	−
Spastic gait	+	+	+	+	+	+	−	−
Trigonocephaly	+	+	+	++	+	+	+	+
Hydrocephalus (CT)	+	+	+	++	++	++	+	+

Figure. The pedigree tree and clinical features of affected members in this family. Arrow indicates the proband. Black circles and squares have hydrocephalus with trigonocephaly. There is no consanguinity.

relation to the adjacent skull bones, we proposed that trigonocephaly and the venous abnormalities are genetically determined developmental errors, resulting on the communicating hydrocephalus in this family members. (Brain and Nerve 38: 917–923, 1986)

Key words: Hereditary communicating hydrocephalus, Trigonocephaly, Dementia

III)   Symptomatology

The Normal Range of the Cerebral Atrophy During Aging:
The statistical analysis of 500 normal subjects

Kazuya Nagata, Norihiko Basugi, Takanori Fukushima, Toshiro Tango, Tsuguchika Kaminuma, Isamu Suzuki, and Shiusuke Kurashina

Department of Neurosurgery, Saitama Medical Center, Saitama Medical School, Kawagoe, Saitama, Japan

A new method of discriminating pathological cerebral atrophy from physiological atrophy during aging is reported. The authors previously reported a new method, *i.e.* pixel counting method, to measure the degree of cerebral atrophy from CT scan (CCR; CSF-cranial ratio). In order to determine the normal range of physiological cerebral atrophy during aging, five hundred normal subjects were studied with this pixel counting method. The scatter plots of the CCR values by age suggested that the CCR values remain relatively constant until about 50 years of age, but thereafter increase with a wider dispersion which appears to be proportional to age. From this findings, the normal range of physiological cerebral atrophy was estimated by means of the maximum likelihood method as follows; Age<48: $0.32<CCR<5.78$, Age>48: $0.068t-2.944<CCR<0.368t-11.884$. Since we previously proposed a simple formula for the calculation of CCR from the comparison of the conventional linear measurement method with pixel counting method, pathological cerebral atrophy is easily detectable using this formula and the determined normal range.

(Brain and Nerve 38: 1019–1025, 1986)

Key words: Cerebral atrophy, Aging, Quantitative analysis, CT scan

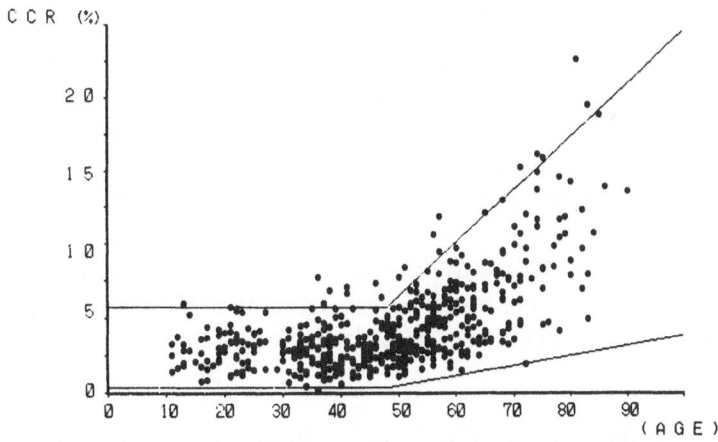

Figure. Scatter plots between age and CCR on 500 normal subjects. The normal range calculated using maximum likelihood method is displayed.

Reversal of Fixed Pupils after Spontaneous Intraventricular Hemorrhage with Secondary Acute Hydrocephalus:
Report of two cases treated with early ventriculostomy

M. Seth Hochman

Department of Neurology, University of Miami School of Medicine, Miami, Florida, USA

The development of fixed pupils in a comatose patient is such an ominous prognostic sign that its occurrence usually signifies a fatal outcome. However, in the 1970s a few reports appeared that documented recovery from fixed pupils resulting from both compressive and noncompressive lesions of the midbrain. The former group consisted primarily of a small number of patients with intracerebral hematomas secondary to ruptured cerebral aneurysms and postoperative and traumatic extradural and subdural hematomas who recovered after prompt neuropharmacological and neurosurgical intervention. The second group, without mass lesions and including less than a dozen cases, contained mainly patients who developed fixed pupils and coma after operations for intracranial aneurysms. Much more recently, Van Gijn *et al.* reported reversal of small nonreactive pupils within 1 to 2 days of early ventriculostomy in five patients with acute hydrocephalus secondary to aneurysmal subarachnoid hemorrhage (1985). We now describe an additional case of a middle-aged hypertensive man with spontaneous subarachnoid and intraventricular hemorrhage in whom rapid reversal of fixed pupils, complete external 3rd nerve opthalmoplegia, and coma occurred after ventriculoperitoneal shunting for secondary acute hydrocephalus. We further report a 71-year-old hypertensive man with spontaneous primary intraventricular hemorrhage in whom rapid reversal of fixed pupils, complete external 3rd nerve ophthalmoplegia, and coma occurred after ventricular drainage of secondary acute obstructive hydrocephalus. In contradistinction to our first patient and the five cases of Van Gijn *et al.*, in this second patient multiple computed tomography (CT) brain scans did not reveal evidence of subarachnoid (or intraparenchymal) hemorrhage. Therefore, the development of fixed pupils and coma in this second case could not be attributed to midbrain vasospasm from subarachnoid hemorrhage. Rather, as was suggested by the rapid improvement after shunting in our first case, the reversal of fixed pupils, complete external 3rd nerve ophthalmoplegia, and coma in this second case was clearly the result of ventricular drainage of acute obstructive hydrocephalus. Cases such as the present ones are unsettling in terms of the comment they make with regard to the usually reliable prognostic value of fixed pupils. Nonetheless, it is important to report such cases in order to delineate which patients with this important clinical sign may benefit from aggressive management.

(Neurosurgery 18: 777–780, 1986)

Key words: Acute hydrocephalus, Fixed pupils, Reversal, Ventriculostomy

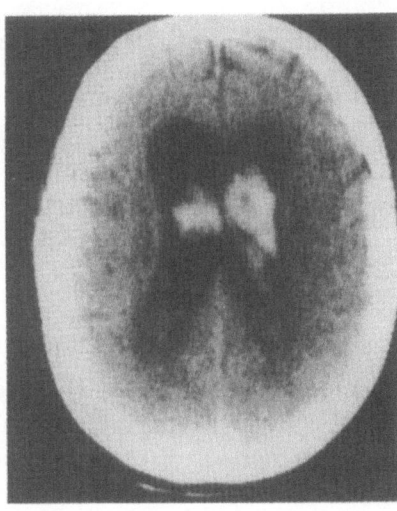

Figure. CT scan of the brain without contrast infusion on admission. Note the presence of intraventricular blood without subarachnoid or intraparenchymal hemorrhage.

Paraplegia Caused by Coarctation of the Aorta and Hydrocephalus

William M. Chadduck, Steven L. Cathey, Anne T. Gearhart, Lillian Cavin, and Charles M. Glasier

Arkansas Children's Hospital; and University of Arkansas for Medical Sciences, Little Rock, Arkansas, USA

A patient with untreated coarctation of the aorta as well as shunt-dependent hydrocephalus developed paraplegia when shunt malfunction resulted in a cerebrospinal fluid pressure greater than 560 mm of water. Improvement followed shunt revision. It is proposed that the unique combination of mechanisms compromised spinal cord perfusion pressure to a critically low level. The low arterial pressure distal to the coarctation of the aorta in combination with an extremely high intraspinal pressure, resulted in a spinal cord perfusion pressure substantially less than 50 mm of mercury, a level quite compatible with spinal cord ischemia. Although the occurrence of aortic coarctation and hydrocephalus is uncommon, the case reemphasizes the concept of an effect of hydrocephalus on spinal cord perfusion pressure and raises the question of a progression of neurologic deficits in some patients having spina bifida complex based on decreased spinal cord perfusion pressure associated with shunt malfunctions. (Child's Nerv Syst 2: 162–164, 1986)

Key words: Paraplegia, Aortic coarctation, Hydrocephalus

Cyst of the Septum Pellucidum Presenting as Hemiparesis

Nobuhiko Aoki

Department of Neurosurgery, Tokyo Metropolitan Fuchu Hospital, Tokyo, Japan

Cysts of the septum pellucidum have been observed with high incidence. After the advent of computed tomography, diagnosis of the cyst has been more easily achieved. However, reports on cysts of the septum pellucidum causing neurological manifestations are extremely rare in the literature; to my knowledge, only two single case reports have been published since introduction of computed tomography scan. An 11-year-old boy with Down syndrome is presented who suffered progressive hemiparesis on the left for a period of 5 years. Computed tomography demonstrated a large cyst of the septum pellucidum and a calcified spot in the head of caudate nucleus on the right (*Figure*). By penetrating the cyst wall to create a communication into the lateral ventricle, shrinkage of the cyst and improvement of the hemiparesis were obtained. The pathogenesis of the hemiparesis was presumed to be attributed to circulatory compromise in the deep cerebral veins, secondary to the cyst.

(Child's Nerv Syst 2: 326–328, 1986)

Key words: Cyst, Septum pellucidum, Hemiparesis, Deep cerebral veins

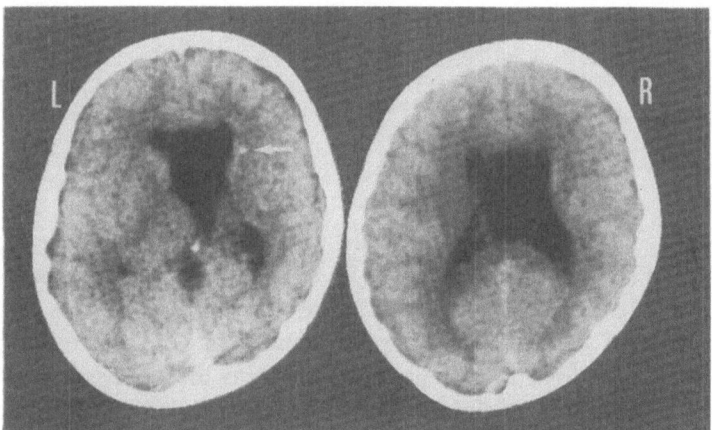

Figure.   Preoperative computed tomography scans, demonstrating a large cyst of the septum pellucidum and a calcified spot in the head of the right caudate head (*arrow*). Both lateral ventricles appear to be displaced laterally. The right thalamus is abnormally small.

IV) Diagnostic Procedures

CT and CT Cisternography
NMR · Positron CT
Ultrasonography and Doppler

The Value of Immediate Post-Operative Routine CT Related to Uncomplicated Ventricle Drainage in Childhood Hydrocephalus

Johan S.H. VLES,[1] Paul CASAER,[1] Jan LODDER,[2] and Christiaan PLETS[3]

Departments of [1]Pediatrics and [3]Neurology and Neurosurgery, University Hospital Gasthuisberg, Leuven, Belgium; [2]Department of Neurology, St. Annadal Hospital, University of Limburg, Maastricht, The Netherlands

Retrospectively we assessed the value of routine postoperative CT scans in 113 children shunted for hydrocephalus. Of the 165 routine CT scans 13 showed fortuitous findings (=8%) with a change in treatment accompanied by questionable benefits in only 2 (=1.3%). Therefore we suggest that post-operative CT should not be performed as a routine examination but only on clinical grounds. (Brain Dev 8: 552–553, 1986)

Key words: Hydrocephalus in childhood, Brain CT, Post-operative follow-up

Magnetic Resonance Demonstration of Normal CSF Flow

John L. SHERMAN and Charles M. CITRIN

Magnetic Imaging of Washington, Chevy Chase, MD, USA

The magnetic resonance (MR) imaging appearance and incidence of flowing cerebrospinal fluid (CSF) in the brain were investigated. The MR scan of 46 randomly selected patients with normal examinations were retrospectively reviewed. All patients were studied using both T_2-weighted and T_1-weighted spin-echo pulse sequences. Thirty-one patients (67%) had decreased intensity in the aqueduct of Sylvius on the T_2-weighted images when compared with the intensity of CSF in the lateral ventricles. This was termed the CSF flow-void sign. The feature was present in the caudal fourth ventricle in 15 patients (32%) and in the third ventricle in two patients (4%) on T_2-weighted scans. It was seen in only 13% of patients on T_1-weighted scans. It is believed the CSF flow-void sign represents pulsatile CSF flow. Its recognition is important because it explains the inhomogeneity in the appearance of the CSF, which could be confused with pathologic processes. It is valuable in the routine evaluation of MR examinations since it reflects CSF circulatory dynamics. (AJNR 7: 3–6, 1986)

Key words: MRI, CSF pulsations, CSF flow-void sign, Aqueduct of Sylvius

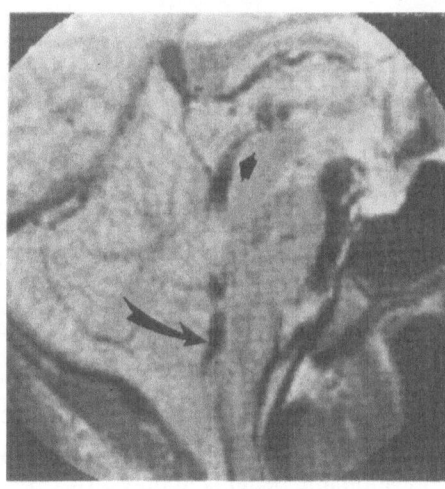

Figure. T$_1$-weighted midline sagittal section in a normal subject. Note CSF flow-void sign due to pulsatile CSF in the aqueduct (*small arrow*) and foramen of Magendie (*curved arrow*).

Magnetic Resonance Demonstration of Altered Cerebrospinal Fluid Flow by Obstructive Lesions

John L. SHERMAN, Charles M. CITRIN, Bruce J. BOWEN, and Raymond E. GANGAROSA

Magnetic Imaging of Washington, Chevy Chase, MD, USA

We investigated the MR imaging appearance of flowing cerebrospinal fluid (CSF) in the brain in the presence of obstructive lesions of the ventricular pathways. The pulsatile movement of CSF through the ventricular system is seen as an area of low signal intensity that has been termed the CSF flow-void sign (CFVS). This is best appreciated in areas of narrowing within the ventricular system; that is, the aqueduct of Sylvius, foramen of Magendie, and interventricular foramina. MR studies of 27 patients with lesions affecting the ventricular pathways were reviewed for the presence of the CFVS. Single-echo T$_1$-weighted and T$_2$-weighted multisection techniques were used in all cases. The CFVS was always seen more prominently on the T$_2$-weighted images. The presence of the CFVS indicated patency of the ventricular pathway in which it was identified. The absence of the CFVS in the presence of hydrocephalus indicated that a possible obstructive lesion was present, but it did not directly indicate the level of the obstruction. The CFVS was absent in the aqueduct of Sylvius in 13 patients with obstruction or stenosis of the aqueduct, but it was also absent in one patient with a colloid cyst of the interventricular foramina. In three patients with preoperative and postoperative MR, the CFVS was seen in the area of interest only after resection of the obstructing lesion. We concluded that the presence of the CFVS is a useful indicator of the patency of the ventricular pathway in which it is seen. The absence of the CFVS at a location in which it is normally seen may indicate the presence of an obstruction, but it must be correlated with other signs to be interpreted correctly.

(AJNR 7: 571–579, 1986)

Key words: MRI, Aqueductal stenosis, Obstructive hydrocephalus, CSF pulsations, CSF flow-void sign

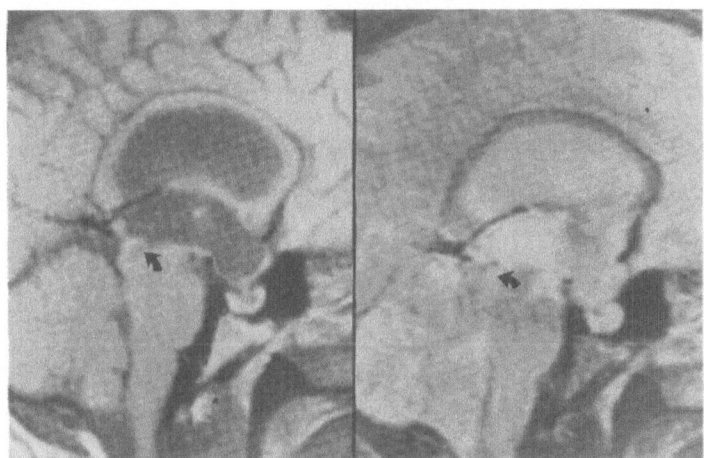

Figure. Aqueductal stenosis. T_1-weighted and T_2-weighted midline sagittal images. Rostral aqueduct is visualized (*curved arrow*) but note absence of CSF flow-void sign in aqueduct indicating obstruction of pulsatile CSF movement through aqueduct. Lateral and third ventricles are dilated, fourth ventricle is small.

The MR Appearance of CSF Flow in Patients with Ventriculomegaly

John L. Sherman, Charles M. Citrin, Raymond E. Gangarosa, and Bruce J. Bowen

Magnetic Imaging of Washington, Chevy Chase, MD, USA

The purpose of this study was to investigate the MR imaging appearance of mobile CSF in the ventricular system in patients with ventriculomegaly caused by brain atrophy and extraventricular obstructive hydrocephalus. Pulsatile CSF often has decreased intensity relative to less mobile areas of CSF, particularly on T_2-weighted scans. At times, the flow-related signal dropout causes striking heterogeneity in the appearance of CSF. This has been termed the CSF flow-void sign (CFVS) and is most likely caused by spin-phase shifts and time-of-flight effects created as a result of CSF turbulence and increased velocity of CSF pulsatile flow. The effect is most pronounced in areas where a larger volume of CSF moves throuth a smaller channel or foramen, such as the aqueduct of Sylvius or foramen of Magendie. The scans of 40 patients with ventriculomegaly caused by brain atrophy or extraventricular obstructive hydrocephalus were reviewed for the presence of the CFVS. All patients had the CFVS in the aqueduct of Sylvius on T_2-weighted spin-echo sequences. The sign was present in the fourth ventricle in 96%, in the third ventricle in 70%, in the foramen of Magendie in 65–77%, and in the foramina of Monro in 33%. The sign was more pronounced in patients with larger ventricles but could not be used to differentiate patients with brain atrophy from those with extraventricular obstructive hydrocephalus.

(AJNR 7: 1025–1031, 1986)

Key words: MRI, CSF pulsations, CSF flow-void sign, Aqueduct of Sylvius

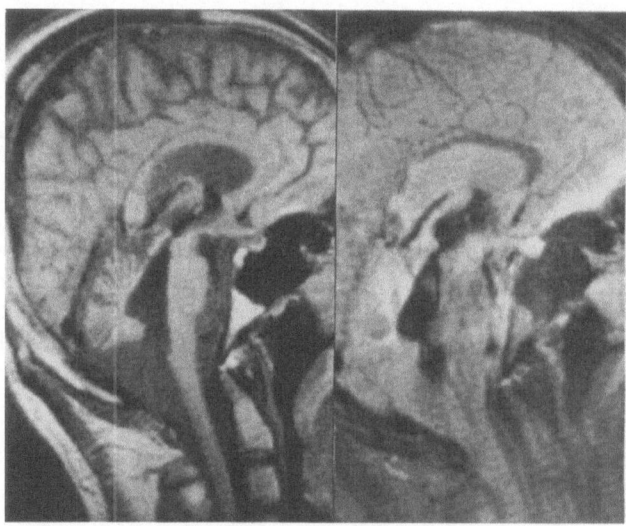

Figure. T_1-weighted and T_2-weighted midline sagittal images in patient with vermian hypoplasia and post-traumatic extraventricular obstructive hydrocephalus. Note markedly hypointense appearance of CSF (CSF flow-void sign) in posterior third ventricle, aqueduct and fourth ventricle compared to CSF in lateral ventricle.

The MR Appearance of CSF Pulsations in the Spinal Canal

John L. Sherman, Charles M. Citrin, Raymond E. Gangarosa, and Bruce J. Bowen

Magnetic Imaging of Washington, Chevy Chase, MD, USA

We investigated the MR appearance and incidence of low-signal areas within the CSF of the spinal canal. Nonuniform areas of decreased signal intensity in intracranial CSF have been named the CSF flow-void sign (CFVS) and appear to be due to spin dephasing secondary to pulsatile CSF motion. Similar areas are seen in the spinal canal. The MR scans of 50 randomly selected patients, constituting a total of 63 spinal studies, were reviewed. There were 27 cervical, 16 thoracic, and 20 lumbar spine examinations. All patients were studied using T_2-weighted and T_1-weighted spin-echo pulse sequences. T_2-weighted images were done with sufficiently long TE and TR to cause the CSF to appear hyperintense compared with brain and spinal cord tissue. Two patients with enlarged spinal canals and two patients with syringomyelia were also included to illustrate the appearance of prominent CSF pulsations.

The CFVS was identified on T_2-weighted scans in the cervical spinal canal in nine patients (33%), in the thoracic spinal canal in one patient (6%), and in the lumbar spinal canal in 2 patients (10%). The CFVS was prominent in two patients with enlarged CSF spaces and was also seen in the intramedullary cavity of the patients with syringomyelia.

The CFVS could obscure small dural lesions and, in some instances, simulate enlarged vessels. Recognition of the spinal CFVS is important to avoid the incorrect diagnosis of intraspinal lesions.   (AJNR 7: 879–884, 1986)

Key words: MRI, Spinal subarachnoid space, CSF pulsations, CSF flow-void sign

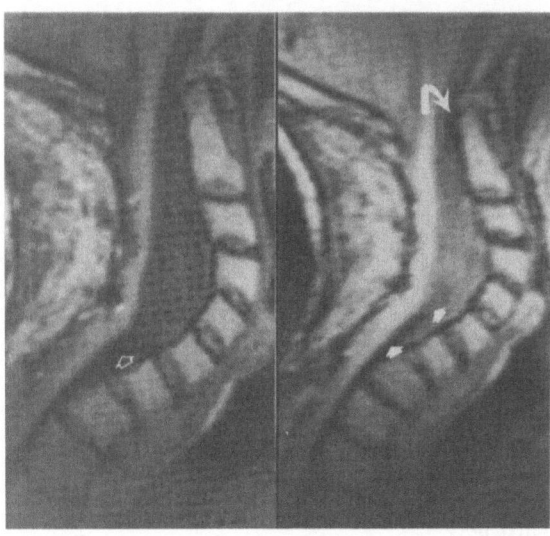

Figure. Enlarged cervical spinal canal from extensive laminectomy. Proton-weighted and T_2-weighted sagittal images. Note heterogeneous appearance of CSF. Hypointense areas (CSF flow-void sign) (*arrows*) due to pulsatile CSF movement are most prominent on T_2-weighted images.

The MR Appearance of Syringomyelia: New observations

John L. SHERMAN, A.J. BARKOVICH, and Charles M. CITRIN

Magnetic Imaging of Washington, Chevy Chase, MD, USA

Fifty-eight patients with spinal cord cavities were studied with MR imaging. Patients were separated into four groups, and the appearance of the cavities were compared. There were 24 patients (41.4%) with communicating syringomyelia (associated with the Chiari I malformation). Sixteen patients (27.6%) had post-traumatic syringomyelia, nine patients (15.5%) had associated tumors, and nine patients (15.5%) had idiopathic syringomyelia. The characteristics of each syrinx, the spinal cord, and the appearance of the cerebellar tonsils were analyzed on T_2- and T_1-weighted images. There is a striking similarity in the appearance of many syrinx cavities regardless of the cause.

Characteristics that were found in some patients in every group included areas of increased intensity on T_2-weighted images, the presence of the CSF flow-void sign (CFVS) in the syrinx cavity, eccentric cavities, "beaded" cavities, and cord enlargement. Tonsillar ectopia alone does not indicate that a syrinx is of the "communicating" type, since it was present in two of

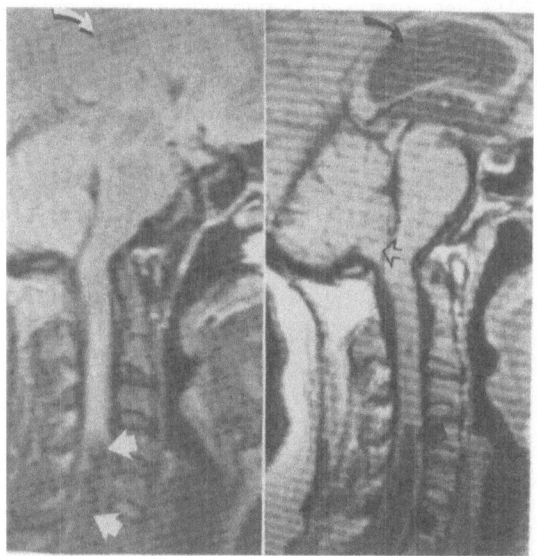

Figure.   Syringomyelia. T_2-weighted and T_1-weighted sagittal images. Lateral ventricles are enlarged (*curved arrows*). The odontoid is deformed and there is cerebellar tonsillar dysplasia (*open arrow*) and spinal cord cavitation (*arrows*). Note hyperintensity of the rostral spinal cord due to gliosis. Also note hypointensity of pulsatile fluid in the syrinx cavity on T_2-weighted images (*white arrows*) compared to "bright" CSF in lateral ventricle.

16 patients (13%) with trauma and in two of five patients (40%) with tumors. T_1-weighted images were most useful in evaluating the anatomic characteristics of the syrinx and the cerebellar tonsils. Most syrinx cavities involved the cervicothoracic junction. The average length was between five and nine vertebral segments (depending on category) but varied between on and 20 vertebral segments. T_2-weighted images revealed areas of increased intensity in the spinal cord in 13 patients without tumors. Two of these cases were shown to represent gliosis on histopathologic review. The CFVS was present in the syrinx cavities of 23 patients (40%), probably reflecting pulsatile movements of the syrinx fluid. It has been proposed that such movements are a cause of syrinx propagation, and the observation of the CFVS may have prognostic significance. The development and progression of the FVS was documented in serial MR examinations in one patient over an 18-month period. The theories of syrinx development and propagation are reviewed.   (AJNR 7: 985–995, 1986)

Key words: MRI, Syringomyelia, CSF pulsations

Flowing Cerebrospinal Fluid in Normal and Hydrocephalic States:
Appearance on MR images

William G. Bradley, Jr.,[1] Keith E. Kortman,[1] and Brian Burgoyne[2]

[1]MR Imaging Laboratory, Huntington Medical Research Institutes; and [2]Department of Radiology, Huntington Memorial Hospital, Pasadena, CA, USA

The signal intensity of the cerebrospinal fluid (CSF) in the cerebral aqueduct and lateral ventricles on magnetic resonance (MR) images was evaluated in 16 healthy individuals and in 32 patients with various forms of hydrocephalus (20 with chronic communicating or "normal pressure" hydrocephalus (NPH), seven with acute communicating hydrocephalus, and five with hydrocephalus ex vacuo (atrophy). The low signal intensity frequently observed in the cerebral aqueduct is believed to reflect the pulsatile motion of CSF which is related to the cardiac cycle. While this "aqueductal flow void phenomenon" can be observed in healthy individuals, it is most pronounced in patients with chronic communicating hydrocephalus; is less evident in patients with acute communicating hydrocephalus; and is least evident in patients with atrophy. Ventricular compliance is known to be essentially normal in atrophy; mildly decreased in acute communicating hydrocephalus; and severely decreased in NPH. The degree of aqueductal signal loss is believed to reflect the velocity of the pulsatile CSF motion, which in turn depends on the relative ventricular compliance and surface area.
                                                           (Radiology 159: 611–616, 1986)

Key words: CSF flow, Hydrocephalus, NPH

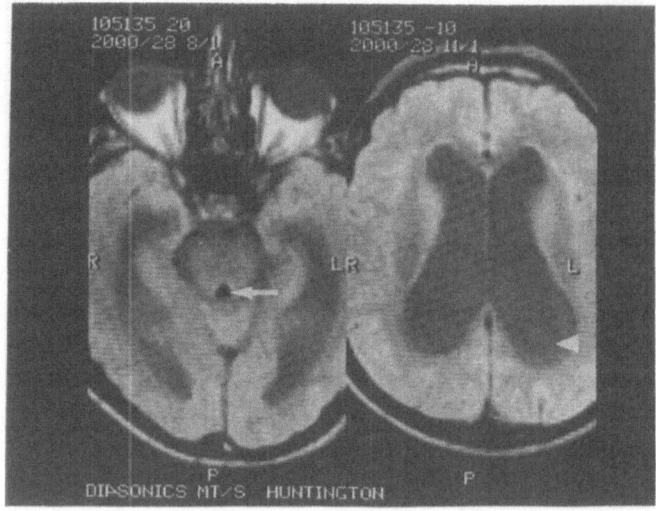

Figure. Aqueductal flow void sign in patient with clinical NPH. Greater signal loss (*arrow*) is noted in aqueduct than in lateral ventricles (*arrowhead*) because of pulsatile flow of CSF. Note other MR findings in NPH: ventricles dilated out of proportion to enlarged cortical sulci, smooth periventricular rim of increased intensity, and absence of focal periventricular lesions (which indicate deep white matter infarction)
(TR [repetition time]=2.0 sec, TE [echo time]=28 msec).

A Quantitative Index of Ventricular and Extra-Ventricular Intracranial CSF Volumes Using MR Imaging

Barrie R. Condon, James Patterson, David J. Wyper, Donald M. Hadley, Graham M. Teasdale, Robin Grant, Alistair Jenkins, Peter Macpherson, and Jack Rowan

Magnetic Resonance Unit, Institute of Neurological Sciences, Southern General Hospital, Govan Road, Glasgow, Scotland

A new technique is described that utilizes a novel magnetic resonance pulse sequence to provide a quantitative index both for ventricular and, for the first time, extra-ventricular intracranial CSF volumes. The pulse sequence is a combination of a null-point inversion recovery sequence with a 4 echo Carr-Purcell read (total echo time=400 ms), which produces a contrast between CSF and other brain tissue of better than 200: 1. A series of experiments was performed on phantoms representing CSF filled ventricles and sulci over a wide range of volume values, and it was found that the standard deviation of differences between true and estimated values was 3.9% for ventricles, 4.6% for total cranial CSF and 7.9% for CSF within the sulci. Normal volunteer reproducibility studies revealed corresponding standard deviations of less than 5.5%. Using the technique to produce absolute estimates of CSF volumes in normal subjects and patients produced results in good agreement with previously published autopsy studies. The total MRI acquisition time is only 10.6 minutes. The technique has wide neurological and neurosurgical applicability particularly in terms of differential diagnosis and as an objective monitor of therapy or progression in such conditions as atrophy, hydrocephalus and benign intracranial hypertension. *Table* is a summary of the most recent work performed on patients suffering from various hydrocephalic conditions. The most significant parameter in differentiating between the various hydrocephalic states and dementia appears to be the ratio of ventricular to cortical sulcal CSF volumes. (J Comput Assist Tomogr 10: 784–792, 1986)

Key words: Cerebrospinal fluid, Volume, Volume determination, Magnetic resonance imaging

Table. Summary of latest work by Grant, R., Condon, B., and Teasdale, G. presented at the Intracranial Pressure and Brain Injury 7th International Symposium, Ann Arbor, 1988 (Abstracts in press)

Subjects	Number of Patients	Ventricular / Cortical Sulcal — CSF Volume
Normal subjects	25	<0.25
Acute obstructive hydrocephalus	5	0.30–>1.0
Chronic obstructive hydrocephalus	5	>0.9
Dementia	12	<0.31
Normal pressure hydrocephalus	14	0.34–>1.0

Observation of CSF Pulsatile Flow on MRI: The signal void phenomenon and its relation to intracranial pressure

Shigeki OHARA, Takashi MATSUMOTO, and Hajime NAGAI

Department of Neurosurgery, Nagoya City University, Nagoya, Japan

In a retrospective study of the MR images of 289 neurosurgical patients, loss of signal intensity (the signal void phenomenon) of cerebrospinal fluid in the mesencephalic aqueduct was observed in 77 patients. This signal void phenomenon (SVP) was seen most frequently in patients suffering from communicating hydrocephalus (10 of 14), less frequently in patients with supratentorial tumors (7 of 50), and not at all in patients with noncommunicating hydrocephalus (none of 9). Eight of 19 patients with infratentorial lesions who did not demonstrate the SVP preoperatively, developed it after suboccipital craniectomy.

It is known that CSF in the cranial cavity flows toward the spinal CSF space in a to and fro manner in response to pulsations of the brain. The velocity of this flow is faster in the narrower parts in the ventricular system such as the aqueduct, Monro's foramen and the fourth ventricle. The SVP reflects CSF pulsatile flow forced out of the intracranial space into the intraspinal space by the brain's pulsations.

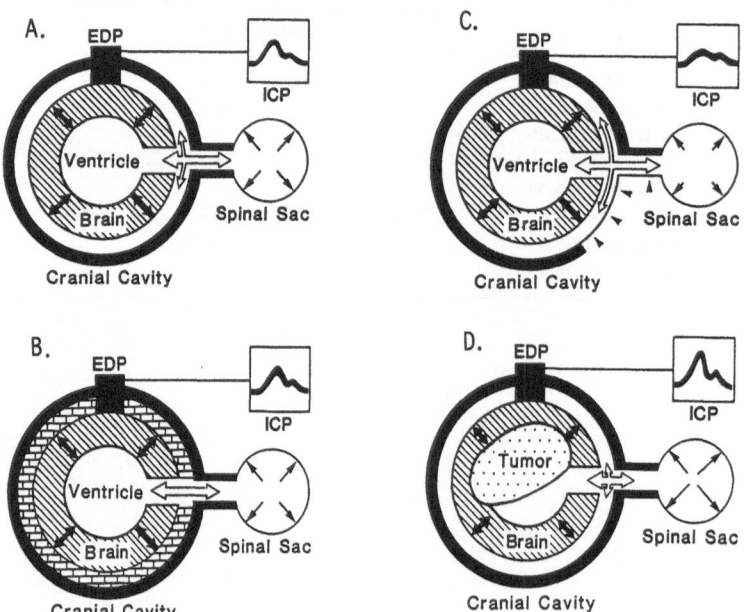

Figure. Hydrodynamics of CSF : Intracranial CSF flows toward the spinal CSF space in a to and fro manner, responding to pulsations of brain parenchyma (**A**). The magnitude of CSF pulsation is changed variously in following conditions: subarachnoid hemorrhage (**B**), craniectomy (**C**) and intracranial hypertension (**D**).

The SVP was observed frequently in the MRI of patients with communicating hydrocephalus who showed normal intracranial mean pressure (ICMP) and normal pulse pressure (PP), whereas the SVP was observed rarely in patients with high ICMP and high PP, such as those with a supratentorial tumor.

The SVP may reflect the capacity of the craniospinal cavity to buffer pressure changes in it. It may be possible to differentiate normal intracranial pressure from high PP by detection of the SVP in CSF in the ventricular system.

(Annual Report of the Research Committee of "Hydrocephalus," The Ministry of Health and Welfare of Japan, 1986: 143–150, 1987)

Key words: Cerebrospinal fluid flow dynamics, Intracranial pressure, Magnetic resonance imaging, Signal void phenomenon

Periventricular Hyperintensity as Seen by Magnetic Resonance: Prevalence and significance

Robert D. Zimmerman, Cynthia A. Fleming, Benjamin C. P. Lee, Leslie A. Saint-Louis, and Michael D. F. Deck

New York Hospital-Cornell University Medical Center, Department of Radiology, New York, NY, USA

Periventricular hyperintensity (PVH) was identified on long TR/intermediate TE (1500/90) scans. PVH was encountered on these images in patients with white matter disease (*e.g.* multiple sclerosis) caused by focal demyelination and in hydrocephalic patients due to transependymal absorption of CSF. A review of 365 consecutive studies demonstrated that PVH is present in most patients (93.5%) regardless of diagnosis. The extent of PVH was divided into five patterns for further evaluation. Grade 0: no PVH; Grade I–discontinuous PVH with small foci of hyperintensity at the angles of the frontal and occipital horns; Grade II–a continuous pencil-thin rim of hyperintensity noted around the lateral ventricles; Grade III–a thicker halo of hyperintensity with smooth lateral borders and; Grade IV–a thick irregular halo of PVH. Mild PVH (Grades I-II) was seen in patients with no other evidence of intracranial pathology and is a normal finding that should not be considered indicative of either demyelinating disease or hydrocephalus. Extent of PVH in these patients is age-related (see *Figure A*). More extensive and severe PVH is associated with intracerebral pathology but the finding is often nonspecific (see *Figure B*). Mild periventricular edema from hydrocephalus is impossible to differentiate from PVH seen in patients with multiple white matter lesions or from the degree of PVH seen in normal elderly patients. Thus, the pattern of PVH has proven to be of limited value in the clinical assessment of hydrocephalic patients. We believe that PVH is a reflection of normal flow of water from the brain interstitium towards and into the ventricular system. Interstitial water is removed from the brain via the ventricles as CSF. In many pathologic conditions (*e.g.* infarction, trauma, tumor and multiple sclerosis), there is increased interstitial water which in turn produces an increase in PVH as a secondary phenomena. In hydrocephalus, the direction of the flow of water is probably reversed (transependymal absorption of the CSF) but its anatomic configuration is the same as that seen in non-hydrocephalic patients with increased interstitial water.

(AJNR 7: 13–20, 1986)

Key words: MRI, Hydrocephalus, Demyelinating disease, Trauma, Brain neoplasm

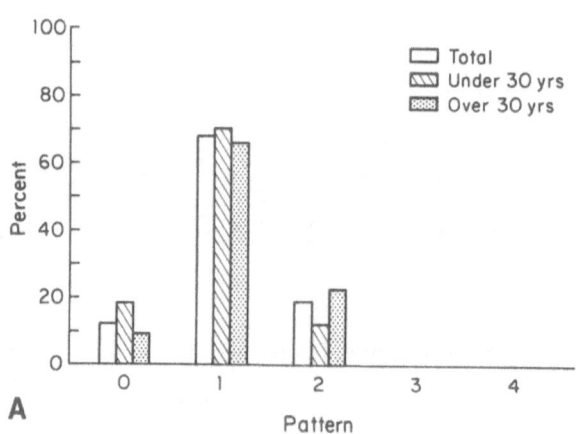

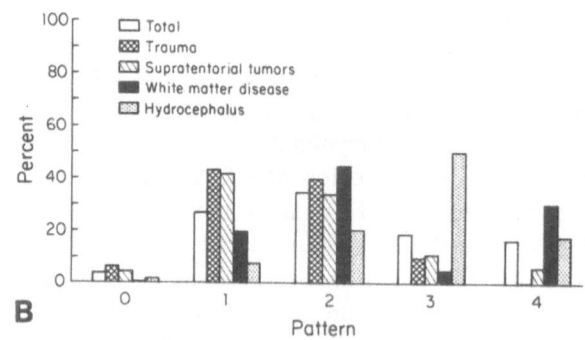

Figure. Incidence of PVH patterns.

(**A**) Otherwise normal group—all patients graded 0-II. PVH grade increases with age. Grade II much more common in patients over 30.

(**B**) In patients with other pathology, all five grades are present. Grade III most typical in hydrocephalus and Grade IV most common in demyelinating disease. Note overlap between groups.

Evaluation of Periventricular Hyperintensity on Magnetic Resonance Images of Normal Brains

Yutaka MAKI, Yuji TOMONO, and Tadao NOSE

Department of Neurosurgery, Institute of Clinical Medicine, University of Tsukuba, Tsukuba, Japan

Periventricular hyperintensity area (PVHI), which appears on magnetic resonance T_2-weighted images in hydrocephalus and other various intracranial lesions, is often observed also in a normal brain. MRI of 239 patients without neurological deficit and intracranial lesion on MRI were evaluated, especially regarding to the incidence of PVHI and an influence of aging. The MR examinations were obtained on a 0.15-T resistive magnet. T_2-weighted images were obtained using spin-echo sequences with TR of 1200 msec and TE of 60 msec.

PVHI was seen in 56 (23.4%) of the 239 patients, but was not found in younger group at all. It began to be seen in some of the patients of the fifth decade, and the higher the age advanced, the more the incidence of PVHI increased. PVHI was observed in the majority of the patients older than 60 years. At first, PVHI tended to appear on the white matter just anterior to the frontal horns and lateral to the bodies followed by extension to the occipital horns with age. Most of the pattern of PVHI in the normal subjects were thin continuous line of high intensity surrounding the ventricles. Though PVHIs were seen like caps of the ventricles in some cases over 70 years of age, a more advanced stage, diffuse white matter abnormality, was not found in the subjects. These stages were given 1, 2 and 3 points respectively, and the PVHI score was defined as the sum of the points on the above-mentioned three sites. The average PVHI score of each generation also increased significantly.

PVHI was thought to be increased local water content, because of not only arteriosclerotic hypoxia but also factors such as focal low myelin content, ependymitis granularis and

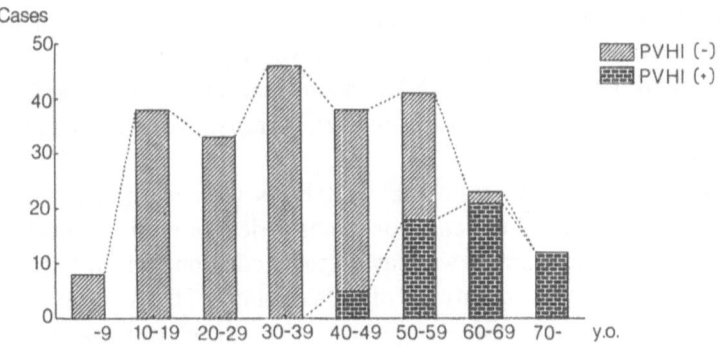

Figure. Age distribution of periventricular hyperintensity (PVHI) on T_2-weighted MR image.

convergence of interstitial fluid flow in this region.

In conclusion, PVHI can be seen on the MRI of a normal brain, and its frequency increases by a factor of aging. Judgment of PVHI in hydrocephalus, therefore, must be made with prudence.

(Annual Report of the Research Committee of "Hydrocephalus," The Ministry of Health and Welfare of Japan, 1986: 151–156, 1987)

Key words: Periventricular hyperintensity, Magnetic resonance image, Normal brain, Aging

Medical Imaging of Fetal Ventriculomegaly

William C. Hanigan, Jack Gibson, Nicholas J. Kleopoulos, Thomas Cusack, George Zwicky, and Robert M. Wright

Departments of Neurosciences, Obstetrics and Gynecology, and Radiology, University of Illinois College of Medicine at Peoria; and Saint Francis Medical Center, Peoria, Illinois, USA

Five cases of fetal ventriculomegaly are described in detail. Following ultrasonography, either computerized tomography or magnetic resonance imaging was used in an attempt to clarify the structural pathology of the ventriculomegaly. Scans were performed at mean gestational age of 32 weeks; all fetuses were delivered at term.

In three infants a precise structural diagnosis was made prior to delivery. In the remainder the cause of the ventriculomegaly could not be established. Two children with aqueductal stenosis and the Arnold Chiari malformation respectively, are meeting developmental milestones; one child with an Arnold Chiari malformation shows delayed motor development. The remaining two patients with a Dandy-Walker malformation and holoprosencephaly expired following delivery.

In summary, these cases demonstrate that in fetuses with ventriculomegaly a definitive radiologic diagnosis should be obtained prior to obstetrical or neurosurgical intervention. A significant proportion of these infants will have associated anomalies or lethal malformations and ancillary imaging will help to clarify the diverse etiology of this clinical entity.

(J Neurosurg 64: 575–580, 1986)

Key words: Fetus, Ventriculomegaly, Computerized tomography, Magnetic resonance imaging

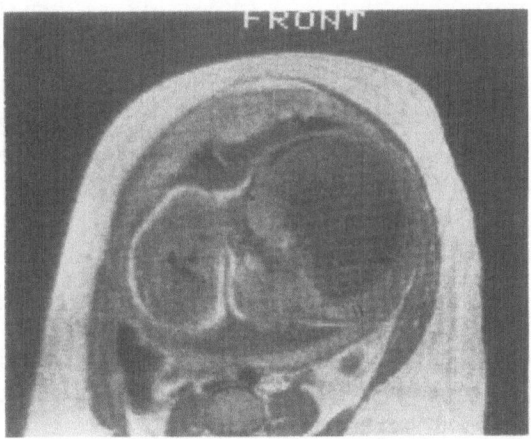

Figure. Axial MRI of a 34 week fetus using a 0.35 Tesla scan with a multislice, multiecho technique. The scan demonstrates an enlarged ventricular system with visualization of the cerebellum (*single arrow*) and midbrain (*asterisk*). The cortical rim (*double arrows*) is seen in this projection.
A prenatal diagnosis of aqueductal stenosis was established.

Statistical Evaluation of Cerebrospinal Fluid Circulation by Radioisotope Cisternography Using SPECT Method: A clinical study

Hiroji KUCHIWAKI, Masato NAGASAKA, Sohshun TAKADA, Hitoshi ISHIGURI, and Naoki KAGEYAMA

Department of Neurosurgery, Nagoya University School of Medicine, Nagoya, Japan

This study is designed to obtain more reliable diagnosis of an impairment of cerebrospinal fluid (CSF) circulation in patients with suspected of hydrocephalus or malfunctions of shunt systems. Such seventeen patients and three control patients (pituitary adenoma; 2, suspected CSF rhinorreal; 1) were included in our study. Twelve male and eight female patients ranged from 18 to 70 year-old (mean 59.5, postoperative follow-up period after a final diagnosis; 2–32 months). Etiologies of the diseases were subarachnoid hemorrhage (4), brain tumor (2), unknown (10), and cryptococcal meningitis(1).
Intrathecal injections of 111-Indium-DTPA (1 mCi) were performed via the ventricle (3) and the lumbar route (17).

Regions of interest (ROI) were selected at Cisterna Magna (CM), Basal Cistern (BC), Cistern of the Lateral Sulcus (CLS), Interhemispheric Cistern (IHC), and the Lateral Ventricle (LV) using axial tomographic images by Single Photon Emission CT (SPECT). The time activity curve of RI (radioisotope) counts at each ROI was plotted and their exponential curves after the peaks were calculated with the least square method (R square$\geqq$0.814). K-values distributed from 0.012 to 0.069 (mean 0.034). A constant (k) of each curve was selected as an indicator of impairment of CSF circulation.

Diagnosis of hydrocephalus was made in a patient showing smaller ks than 0.041 at every ROI except for CM. Thus twelve patients were diagnosed as hydrocephalus. Constants (Ks) in control patients showed larger than 0.041 at BC and LV. Nine of them were treated with ventriculo-peritoneal shunt. Two of them were eliminated as candidates for surgical treatments, because of abnormal psychological behaviours and a recurrence of cancer. One hydrocephalus patient refused surgical treatments.

Various degrees of improvements were observed in seven patients. Subdural hematoma appeared in a patient and the another remained unchanged. Five patients out of our criteria were treated with medications.

The author's results with SPECT seem to be more useful than those by routine static images with a gamma camera.

(Annual Report of the Research Committee of "Hydrocephalus," The Ministry of Health and Welfare of Japan, 1986: 135–142, 1987)

Key words: Cerebrospinal fluid (CSF) circulation, Single photon emission CT (SPECT), Radioisotope

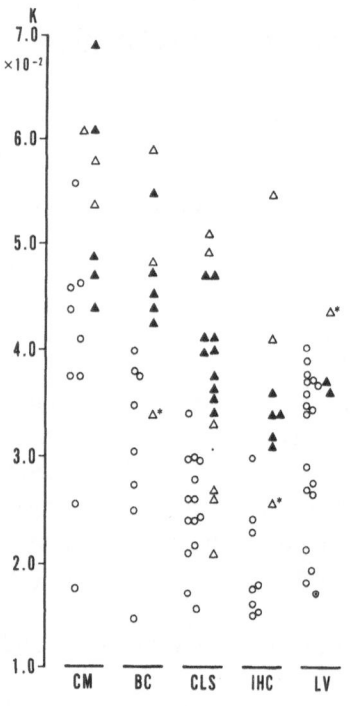

Figure. Graph showing distribution of k value at each ROI. Hydrocephalus group: open circle, control group: closed triangle, open triangles with asterics: case 19 control, a circle including a dot: fourth ventricle of case 12: hydrocephalus. Abbreviations: see text.

Ultrasound Examination in the Detection, Diagnosis and Management of Fetal and Neonatal Intracranial Abnormalities

Yushiro YAMASHITA,[1] Toyojiro MATSUISHI,[1] Yoichiro YAMAGUCHI,[1] Etsuo OTAKI,[1] Takamoto MATSUNAGA,[2] Junji ISHIMATSU,[2] and Teiji HAMADA[2]

Departments of [1]Pediatrics and [2]Obstetrical Gynecology, Kurume University, Kurume, Japan

With the advances in and increased availability of ultrasonography, prenatal diagnosis of an intracranial abnormality is now enabled. Here we report our evaluation of the ultrasonographic detection during pregnancy of intracranial abnormalities in 6 patients, with evaluation of the prenatal diagnosis, management and prognosis.

Method

Between March 1984 and November 1985, 840 high risk pregnant women were admitted to

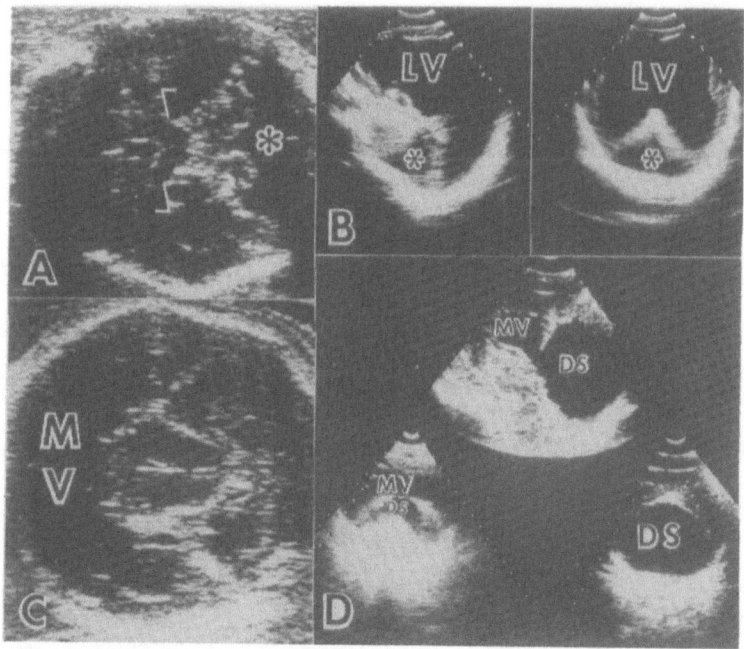

Figure. (**A, B**) Dandy-Walker syndrome
Ultrasonogram at 30 weeks of gestation (**A**) and after birth (**B**).
Lateral ventricular enlargement (Δ, LV) and midline cyst in posterior fossa (*).
(**C, D**) Holoprosencephaly (alobar type)
Ultrasonogram at 31 weeks of gestation (**A**) and after birth (**B**).
Mono ventricle (MV) and dorsal sac (DS).

Kurume University Hospital. Prenatal ultrasound scans were performed after 15 weeks of gestation at 1 month intervals. 239 neonates were admitted to the neonatal intensive care unit and echoencephalography was performed repeatedly after birth. A total of 6 neonates were diagnosed as having an intracranial abnormality detected by ultrasound examination during the prenatal period.

Results and Discussion

The 6 patients with intracranial abnormality involved hydrocephalus with neural tube defect (3), Dandy-Walker syndrome (1), holoprosencephaly (1) and arteriovenous malformation (AVM) of Galen (1). An accurate diagnosis was made prenatally in all except for the case of AVM of Galen, in which the diagnosis was confirmed only postnatally. This correct noninvasive diagnosis of AVM of Galen establishes the efficacy of both two-dimensional echoencephalography and of echocardiography, combined with pulsed Doppler observation. There have been no reports with respect to Doppler echocardiography on cerebral AVM. Our case of AVM of Galen revealed significant diastolic Doppler signal on the aortic arch, which suggests a presence of cerebral A-V fistula. In the 4 patients with hydrocephalus (the 3 patients with neural tube defect and the one with Dandy-Walker syndrome), V-P shunt operation was performed shortly after birth. The prognosis was very poor in 3 patients, with holoprosencephaly (1), AVM of Galen (1), and with hydrocephalus with neural tube defect (1). The prognosis is good in the patient with Dandy-Walker syndrome at 1 year and 6 months of age with now normal psychomotor development.

(No to Hattatsu 18: 326–329, 1986)

Key words: Intracranial abnormality, Ultrasonography, Prenatal diagnosis, Management

Real-time Compound Scanning for Echoencephalography

M. de VLIEGER, W. BAERTS, C. M. LIGTVOET, and J. C. M. VAN DER SLUYS

University Hospital Sophia-Dijkzigt, Erasmus University, Rotterdam, the Netherlands

One-dimensional echoencephalography (A-mode) ultrasound imaging is improved by B-mode scanning methods for two-dimensional cross-sectional pictures of the brain. In 1963 we developed a manual mechanical compound scanning technique, which offered a so-called "Static two-dimensional echoencephalographic image."

To improve cross-sectional echoencephalographic imaging, both mechanical scanning systems with pivoting transducers and multi-element scanning systems were developed with this equipment. Scanning was conducted through the anterior fontanelle.

The ultrasound beam of a real time compound may visualize more reflecting planes than a sector scanning technique. For two-dimensional echencephalographic imaging in newborns a multi-element real-time compound scanner with dynamic focussing was applied. The goal was to get tomographic pictures of the brain in three dimensions.

Method

A 3 MHz transducer with an array of 102 mm consisting of 256 elements is placed on the skull. A switching matrix incorporated in the transducer assembly selects 49 different groups of 64-adjacent elements. Each group is four elements shifted in relation to the preceding one and produces a phased array image of 90°. Overlapping phased array images produce the compound effect. The reflected ultrasound beams can be focussed at elected distances from the probe.

Results

Results of cranial compound scanning with dynamic focussing of a normal brain, hydrocephalic ventricles and an extracranial haemorrhage are reported. An example of dynamic focussing is given. In *Figure a* at 2 cm focussing from the probe shows an indication of gyri, *Figure b* at 4 cm the septum pellucidum, IIIrd ventricle, IVth ventricle and cerebellum, *Figure c* at 6 cm shows a detailed picture of IVth ventricle and cerebellum.

Advantages of real-time compound scanning:

1) Brain structures may be examined in three dimensions.
2) Infants with closed fontanelles may be examined with 3 MHz.

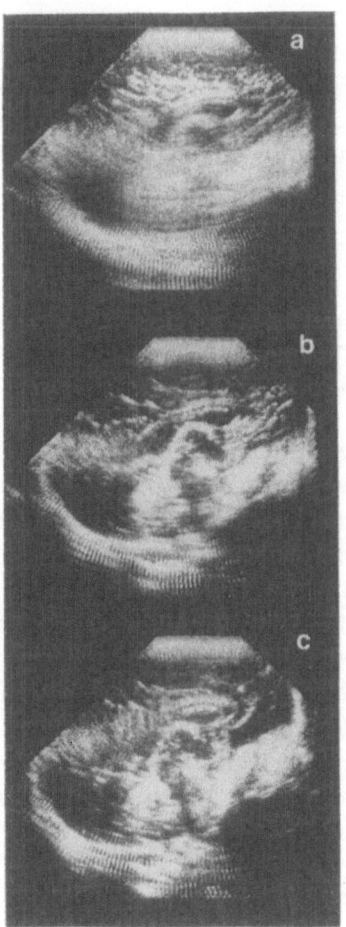

Figure. Sagittal tomography in a normal baby with dynamic focussing of the reflected ultrasound. (**a**) focussing at 2 cm, (**b**) focussing at 4 cm, (**c**) focussing at 6 cm (see text).

3) Dynamic focussing shows circumscribed cerebral abnormalities more exactly.
4) This scanner covers brain structures in a greater area than sector scanning.

(Acta Neurochir 79: 30–34, 1986)

Key words: Ultrasonic scanning technique, Three dimensional pictures, Dynamic focussing

Effects of Hydrocephalus and Increased Intracranial Pressure on Auditory and Somatosensory Evoked Responses

Leslie N. Sutton,[1] Byung-kyu Cho,[2] Jurg Jaggi,[3] Peter M. Joseph,[4] and Derek A. Bruce[5]

[1,2,5]Department of Neurosurgery, Children's Hospital of Philadelphia, [1,3,5]Department of Neurosurgery, University of Pennsylvania School of Medicine, [4]Department of Radiology and Physics and [5]Department of Pediatrics, University of Pennsylvania School of Medicine, Philadelphia, Pennsylvania, and [2]Department of Neurosurgery, College of Medicine, Seoul National University Hospital, Seoul, Korea

Recent studies in human and animal subjects have suggested a relationship between intracranial pressure (ICP) and ventricular dilatatation and multimodality evoked responses which, if substantiated, would be of value to clinical practice as a noninvasive way of assessing the need for shunting in selected patients in whom computed tomography (CT) is not definitive. In an attempt to better define these changes, auditory evoked response (BAER) and somatosensory evoked response (SER) were performed on 16 cats as a base line, after which they were made hydrocephalic by the cisternal injection of kaolin. Nine cats survived, and CT or magnetic resonance scans were performed on them 4 to 6 weeks later. In those animals in which ventricular dilatation was noted, repeat evoked responses were recorded. In the 6 hydrocephalic cats, the ventricle was punctured to measure ICP, which in all cases was less than 5 mm Hg. The lumbar spinal dural sac was then ligated, which resulted in periodic plateau waves up to 75 to 100 mm Hg after 4 to 6 hours, lasting up 10 minutes. In neither group of cats was any change in either BAER or SER observed until preterminally, when ICP was in the range of 75 to 100 mm Hg and cerebral perfusion pressure was compromised. This suggests that the BAER and SER are not sensitive to either ventricular dilatation or intracranial hypertension.

(Neurosurgery 18: 756–761, 1986)

Key words: Evoked response, Hydrocephalus, Increased intracranial pressure, Magnetic resonance imaging

V)   Therapeutic Procedures

Shunt Procedures
Shunt and Shunt Device
Shunt Function (Test)
Shunt Complications

The Value of Multiple Shunt Systems in the Treatment of Nontumoral Infantile Hydrocephalus

G. KAISER

Department of Pediatric Surgery, University Children's Hospital Inselspital, Berne, Switzerland

A multiple shunt system (MSS) has been employed in 9 children with hydrocephalus combined with not or insufficiently communicating CSF or other intracranial fluid filled spaces. The results are used to discuss the reasons for its indication in general and in specific lesions (clinical signs, specific pathology being present, types and results of preoperative work-up examinations), the MSS itself (types of MSS, advantages and disadvantages), its overall value (clinical outcome and types and results of postoperative follow-up examinations) and the problems related to shunt dysfunction in MSS. There arise 4 general indications for a MSS: 1° The uniform drainage of CSF spaces which do not or only insufficiently communicate with each other; 2° The uniforme drainage of CSF and other separate liquid filled intracranial spaces; 3° To obtain an harmonic diminution of enormously dilated CSF or other fluid filled spaces; 4° The use of both sides for shunting in cases with recurrent failures of an unilateral drainage. Specifically a MSS may be applied in post-shunt unilateral hydrocephalus, in trapped lateral ventricles (*e.g.* post-meningitic hydrocephalus), in chronic subdural hematoma, Dandy-Walker syndrome and insolated 4th ventricle hydrocephalus. Supratentorial and posterior fossa cysts are open to discussion for a MSS. The preoperative simultaneous recording of the ICP at different sites is more reliable than

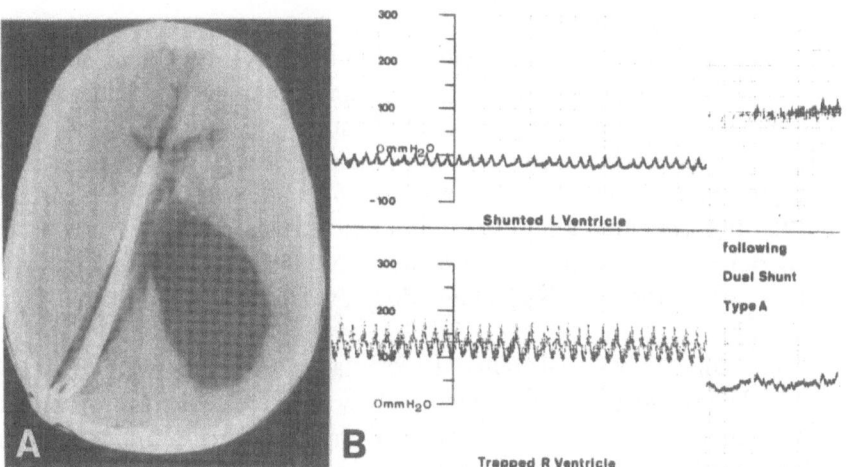

Figure. (A and **B)** Case 7. Hydrocephalus following plexus papilloma surgery. 2 years following implantation of a left ventriculo-peritoneal shunt; trapped right lateral ventricle. Difference of ICP and amplitude of the pulse wave between the right and left lateral ventricle. Pressure equilibrium following a MSS.

the CTT (differences in pressure). The type A shunt (combined drainage of separate spaces with a common valve and distal section) is superior to type B shunt (completely separate shunts) due to a better equilibration of different pressures and a smaller display. The overall value of MSS consists of evenly decreasing CSF and other fluid filled cavities and of an equilibrium of the different ICP's, what can be proved clinically and by CCT and ICP recordings. In possible shunt failure, in addition to these examinations CSF samples of the different drained sites must be tested to discover the precise section of obstruction.

(Child's Nerv Syst 2: 200–205, 1986)

Key words: Multiple shunt systems, Treatment of nontumoral infantile hydrocephalus, Insufficient communication of CSF spaces, Equilibrium of different ICP's

Ventriculosubgaleal Shunt:
An effective CSF drainage in shunt disconnection

S. Constantini,[1] U. Wald,[1] R. Katzenelson,[2] and M. Shalit[1]

[1]Department of Neurosurgery and [2]Department of Anesthesiology, Hadassah University Hospital, Jerusalem, Israel

Von Miculicz (1896) was the first to try internal drainage of the lateral ventricles.[1] He inserted a nail-shaped mass of glass wool into the lateral ventricle and put the end of the drain below the positioned periostal flap. This and other divertion methods have been abandoned in favor of ventriculo-peritoneal shunts.

We describe a 4 years old child with a right ventriculo peritoneal shunt that was disconnected distal to the antisiphon device. The child was asymptomatic except for a huge subcutaneous fluid collection that appeared a few weeks prior to her admission. On CT, a normal sized ventricular system was seen. Abdominal X rays showed the entire Raimondi catheter intra peritoneally. At operation the subgaleal pseudocyst was found to the isolated from the distol shunt tract.

Several factors might have contributed to the lack of symptoms in this patient. The compliance of the pseudocyst was sufficient to allow progressive expansion without an effect on intracranial pressure or ventricular size. It is unlikely that the pseudocyst drained the entire CSF production. Probably the patient retained some CSF absorptive capacity while the cyst functioned as a reservoir for excess fluid. It is also possible that the cyst wall maintained absorptive capacity, similar to the mechanism suggested for sub-temporal decompression in pseudotumor cerebri.[2] This case illustrates a rare complication of shunt proximal disconnection. This progressively enlarging subgaleal pseudocyst was a sufficient CSF draining system. To the best of our knowledge, this entity has not previously been described in the literature.[3] (Child's Nerv Syst 2: 277–278, 1986)

Key words: Ventriculoperitoneal shunt, Shunt malfunction, Subgaleal space, Shunt disconnection

References
1) Miculicz, J.: Beitrag zur pathologie und therapie des hydrocephalus. Mitt. Grenzgeb. Med. Chir., 1: 264, 1896.
2) Bancroft, F.W., Pilcher, C. (eds.): Surgical treatment of the nervous system. Lippincott, Philadelphia, 1946.
3) Choux, M. (ed.): Shunts and problems in shunts. (Monographs in neurological sciences, vol. 8) Karger, Basel, 1982.

Burr Hole Third Ventriculo-cisternostomy:
An unpopular but effective procedure for treatment of certain forms of occlusive hydrocephalus

H. Jaksche and F. Loew

Neurosurgical Clinic of the Saarland University, Homburg/Saar, FRG

Seventy-nine cases of obstructive hydrocephalus treated between 1972 and 1983 by burr hole third ventriculo-cisternostomy have been analysed together with the published literature. There were 80% good results in non-tumoral aqueduct stenosis and in hydrocephalus caused by pineal, posterior third ventricle or basal ganglia tumours.
The results in hydrocephalus caused by dysrhapic malformations or following meningitis as well as in cases which previously had been treated by shunting procedure were unsatisfactory. Such cases therefore should be excluded from third ventriculo-cisternostomy. In the first mentioned cases the patency of the basal cisterns should be verified beforehand by CSF scintigraphy. Only cases with open cisterns should be selected for third ventriculo-cisternostomy. If these selection guidelines are followed good results can be expected in approximately 90%.
Judging from the literature and from our own material the mortality rate is below 1% and the rate of transient neurological deficits about 5%. These complications seem to be avoidable by improved technique.
The alternative methods used in the treatment of obstructive hydrocephalus, viz: ventriculo-cardiac or ventriculo-peritoneal shunting, have an overall complication rate higher than 50%. This comparison leads us to recommend third ventriculo-cisternostomy as

the treatment of choice for properly selected cases of obstructive hydrocephalus.

(Acta Neurochir 79: 48–51, 1986)

Key words: Burr hole, Third ventriculo-cisternostomy, Occlusive hydrocephalus

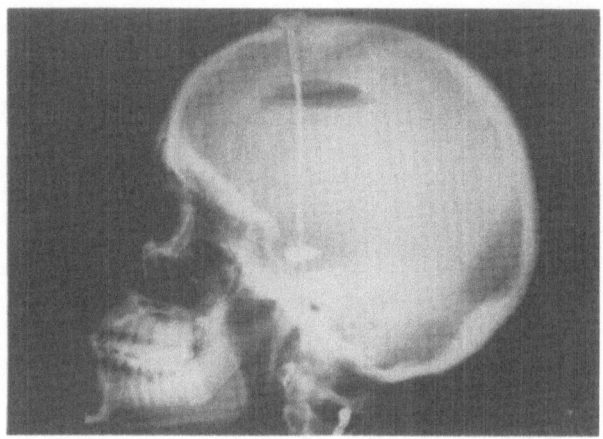

Figure. Burr hole third ventriculo-cisternostomy. The catheter runs through the lateral ventricle, foramen of Monroe and anterior third ventricle just behind the dorsum sellae into the prepontine cistern. Drops of contrast medium are seen within the third ventricle and in the upper cervical subarachnoid space providing proof of the communication between inner and outer CSF spaces.

Lombo-peritoneal Shunt in Non-hydrocephalic Patients: A review of 41 cases

Ph. Bret,[1] J. Huppert,[1] B. Massini,[1] C. Lapras,[2] and G. Fischer[1]

[1]Service de Neurochirurgie C and Faculté Alexis Carrel; and [2]Service de Neurochirurgie B, Hôpital Neurologique de Lyon, France

A population of 41 non-hydrocephalic patients in whom a lumbo-peritoneal shunt (LPS) was inserted for various conditions is reviewed. 19 had persistent cerebro-spinal fluid (CSF) rhinorrhea after cranial injury (14 cases), basal skull surgery (3 cases) or of unknown presumably congenital origin (2 cases). In 15 patients of this group, direct attempts to obliterate the CSF fistula had been unsuccessful. In the 4 others, LPS was employed as a primary treatment of the fistula. 14 had a persistent bulging craniotomy site after operations for intra-cranial tumours (posterior fossa surgery: 7 cases, supra-tentorial surgery:5 cases, open head injury: 2 cases). In this group, LPS was established after failure of repeat lumbar punctures or of external CSF drainage. 3 patients had a so-called benign intra-cranial hypertension (pseudo-tumor cerebri) with persistent headaches and papilledema despite an adequate medical management. 4 patients underwent LPS for syringomyelia. 1 patient presented with a persistent meningocele after removal of a cervical meningioma.

Results:

There was no shunt-related mortality. With a follow-up ranging from 6 years to 6 months, LPS has proved effective in relieving the initial symptoms in 31 patients. In the group of 19 patients treated by this procedure for cranial CSF fistula, 17 showed prompt cessation of rhinorrhea after shunting. In 2 patients of this group, a further intra-cranial approach was needed. Further revision or removal of the shunt was needed on 9 occasions in 8 patients having mechanical or septic shunt-related complications or persistent postural headaches. This report demonstrates the safety of LPS procedure, which has been simultaneously experienced in another group of 146 patients involved with communicating hydrocephalus. Authors' experience demonstrates the variety of the clinical applications of LPS. This technique should be considered in patients requiring a CSF diversion and in whom CT scan shows no or minimal ventricular dilatation. (Acta Neurochir 80: 90–92, 1986)

Key words: Percutaneous lumbo-peritoneal shunt, CSF rhinorrhea, Pseudo-tumour cerebri, CSF shunt

Table.

Diagnosis (+ number of patients)	Aetiology	Previous procedures	Result of LPS	Further procedures
Cranial CSF fistula (19)	traumatic: 14 post-operative: 3 unknown: 2	1 or several direct approaches: 15	cessation of rhinorrhoea: 17	further direct approach needed: 2 shunt revision: 2 shunt removal: 3 (postural headaches: 2 infection: 1)
Pseudo tumour cerebri (3)	contraceptive therapy: 2 unknown: 1	none (conservative therapy)	improvement of papilloedema and headaches in all 3 cases	none
Bulging craniotomy ("meningocele") (14)	posterior fossa surgery: 7 supra-tentorial tumour surgery: 5 head injury (penetrating wound): 2	ventriculo-jugular shunt: 1 ventriculo-peritoneal shunt: 1	prompt resolution of collection 10 failure of LPS: 3 unknown result: 1 death (unrelated to LPS): 2	shunt revision: 1 shunt removal: 3 (postural headaches: 1 failure of LPS: 2) ventriculo-jugular shunt:1
Syringomyelia (4)		cranio-cervical decompressive operation: 2	no significant improvement in the 4 patients	further cranio-cervical decompression needed in 2
Cervical meningocele (1)	post-operative	intra-dural meningioma removal	resolution of fluid collection	none

Symptomatic Progressive Ventriculomegaly in Hydrocephalics with Patent Shunts and Antisiphon Devices

David C. McCullough

Department of Neurosurgery, Children's Hospital National Medical and George Washington University School of Medicine, Washington, District of Columbia, USA

The antisiphon device (ASD) was designed to prevent excessive negative intracranial pressure and overdrainage with cerebrospinal fluid shunts. It is used for prevention of slit ventricles and extreme shunt dependency. The author used the device in 40 children and young adults selectively for the treatment of shunt-produced low pressure headaches or prophylactically for patients judged to be at risk for development of subdural hematomas because of extreme hydrocephalus, fixed head size or tall stature. In 9 of these patients adverse symptoms occurred in spite of shunt patency. Four case reports describe patients 9, 15, 23, and 27 years of age who actually deteriorated after conversion to shunts incorporating ASD's. Typically, deterioration occurred after the patient assumed an erect position. With patients in the horizontal position shunt patency was documented (*Figure*), but computed tomography revealed progressive ventriculomegaly when they were kept erect. Their symptoms disappeared and ventricular size diminished after conversion to proximal medium pressure diaphragm or spring-ball valve systems without ASD's.

Long shunt systems with ASD's require adequate hydrostatic columns to initiate flow when patients are erect. In the author's opinion symptoms develop because of close proximity of antisiphon devices to entry burr holes at ventricular levels. The pressure-flow relationships

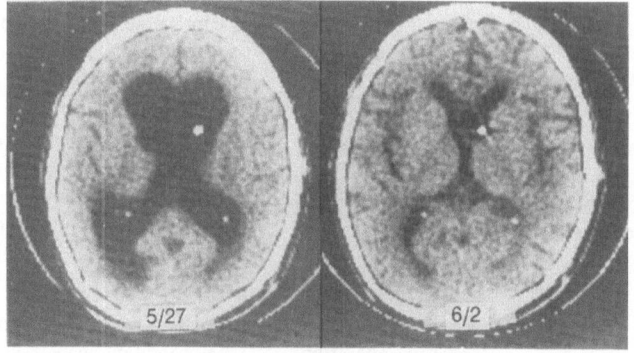

Figure. CT images (*left*) after initial shunt revision and incorporation of ASD in an unconscious patient with marked ventriculomegaly, which responded dramatically to placing the patient in a horizontal position for four days (*right*).

supporting this interpretation were originally described by Fox, Portnoy and Schulte[1] at the time of introduction of the ASD. The greater the negative pressure (attributed to siphoning) inside the shunt the greater the obligatory opening pressure. It is theorized that such symptoms could have been prevented in the author's patients by placing ASD's farther downstream from the cerebral ventricles. (Neurosurgery 19: 617–621, 1986)

Key words: Antisiphon device, Cerebrospinal fluid shunt, Hydrocephalus

Reference
1) Fox, J. L., Portnoy, H. D., Schulte, R. R.: Cerebrospinal fluid shunts: An experimental evaluation of flow rates and pressure values in the antisiphon valve. Surg. Neurol., 1: 299–302, 1973.

Spontaneous Transection of Raimondi Peritoneal Catheter in Twice: A case report with scanning electron microscopic study of transected tube

Tetsuya Sakamoto, Hisashi Kojima, Katsuya Futawatari, and Masayoshi Kowada

Neurosurgical Service, Akita University Hospital, Akita, Japan

A Raimondi peritoneal catheter is employed to avoid the complications arising from the vending of conventional catheters. However, perforation of intraperitoneal organs or spontaneous transection of the catheter has been recently reported. We present a case of spontaneous transection of a Raimondi peritoneal catheter.

A 6-month-old male was admitted to the hospital because of an enlarged head. He had ventriculoperitoneal shunt surgery using Raimondi peritoneal catheter and Dow Corning ventricular catheter for communicating hydrocephalus.

Six months after the operation, however, he suddenly started vomiting and Raimondi peritoneal catheter was found to be spontaneous transected in a peritoneal cavity. Upon restoration of the shunt system, slight retention of serous ascites was noted. A spring wire was stretched and protruded approximately 1 cm from the end of the transected catheter. Scanning electron microscopic examination demonstrated the broken end of the spring wire had cracked and it was suggested that the transection was caused by repetitive exertion of external forces. Replacement with a silicone tube (Dow Corning-Ames type) produced favorable postoperative results.

At the age of 5 year-old, the originally installed Raimondi catheter was again transected on the portion of chest wall. Scanning electron microscopic examination of the broken end of spring wire demonstrated to be dimple caused by forced tension.

All four cases of transection of this catheter so far reported are in children less than 15 years of age. The rapid growth and increased physical activity in childhood are considered to be involved in causing fracture of the catheter.   (*Noshinkei Geka* 14: 1039–1042, 1986)

Key words: Raimondi catheter, Hydrocephalus, Ventriculoperitoneal shunt

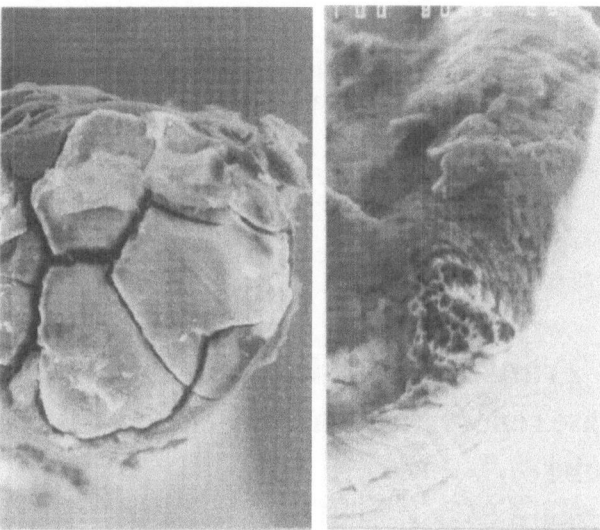

Figure. Scanning electron microscopy demonstrating different findings of broken surface of stainless wire. *left* (first time): the end of the catheter had cracked. *right* (second time): broken surface showed to be dimple.

Management of Obstructive Hydrocephalus Secondary to Posterior Fossa Tumors by Steroids and Subcutaneous Ventricular Catheter Reservoir

Urs D. Schmid and Rolf W. Seiler

Department of Neurosurgery, University-Hospital, Berne, Switzerland

Large tumors in the posterior fossa obstruct the forth ventricle and lead to hydrocephalus resulting in acute or chronic intracranial pressure (ICP). The therapy before tumor removal is therefore always directed toward treatment of the hydrocephalus. In the past, this has traditionally been achieved by the combined use of high dose corticosteroids and ventricular shunting. However, the extensive list of potential complications caused by internal shunts (upward herniation, shunt promoted tumor metastasis, shunt dependency, infections, malfunction) or by external ventricular drainage (infections) strongly speek against their routine use.

In 61 patients (38 adults, 23 children) with surgically treatable tumors, signs and symptoms of rised ICP and obstructive hydrocephalus (incidence see *Table*), the following therapeutic protocol was employed: 1. A high dose of steroids (3 mg/kg/day) was given after diagnosis. 2. A frontal ventricular catheter with a subcutaneous fluid reservoir (Rickham) was inserted within 2–5 days. 3. External ventricular drainage to the reservoir was only attached when ICP during catheter insertion exceeded 30 cm H_2O, the overflow pressure was then kept at 20–25 cm H_2O. 4. Surgery was performed within the next 2–5 days to reopen the CSF pathways. The reservoir was punctured to remove 10–20 m*l* CSF immediately prior to surgery. 5. Internal shunts were inserted only when ICP remained high for 2–4 weeks despite repeated CSF punctures or external ventricular drainage.

With this regimen, 93% of all patients (38 adults, 19 children) remained shunt-free after operation, without fatal complications, the infection rate was 4.9%. Nor the severity of the preoperative signs and symptoms of rised ICP, the ventricular width or the intraventricular pressure measured on occasion of insertion of the ventricular catheter, nor the site and size or the histology of the tumor were found to have prognostic value as to which patients required a shunt after surgery (incidence see *Table*). (J Neurosurg 65: 649–653, 1986)

Key words: Brain tumor, Posterior fossa, Hydrocephalus, Shunt, Glucocorticosteroids

Table. *Post*operative shunt incidence correlated to the incidence of *pre*operative findings (ventricular width, intraventricular pressure, tumor size, signs and symptoms)[1]

Patients	Ventricular width[2]	Intraventricular pressure (cm H_2O)[3]	Size of the tumor[4]	Signs & symptoms	
Adults	40–60% (7/0)	≤20 (11/0)	50–70% (9/0)	Hydrocephalus Triad	(26/0)
n=38	30–39% (14/0)	21–29 (19/0)	30–49% (20/0)	Headache/vomiting	(8/0)
No shunt	20–29% (7/0)	30–50 (8/0)	20–29% (9/0)	Stupor/coma	(4/0)
Children	40–60% (5/1)	≤20 (8/0)	50–70% (11/1)	Hydrocephalus Triad	(16/4)
n=23	30–39% (13/2)	21–29 (8/3)	30–49% (10/2)	Headache/vomiting	(2/0)
4 shunts	20–29% (5/0)	30–50 (7/1)	20–29% (2/1)	Stupor/coma	(5/0)

1. In parentheses: Incidence of pre-operative findings/Incidence of correlated shunt insertion.
2. Ventricular width (tips of the frontal horns) is given as a percentage of the inner diameter of the skull (frontal-horn index, range in normal subjects: 20–30%).
3. Intraventricular pressure at catheter placement after 2–5 days pretreatment with corticosteroids.
4. Size of the tumor is given as percentage of the inner diameter of the posterior fossa.

The Use of Shunting Devices for Cerebrospinal Fluid in Canada

Harold J. Hoffman[1] and May S. M. Smith[2]

[1]Division of Neurosurgery,The Hospital for Sick Children, University of Toronto, Toronto, Ontario; and [2]Clinical Criteria Bureau of Medical Devices, Environmental Health Directorate, Health and Welfare, Ottawa, Ontario, Canada

During the year 1982/1983, 3,162 shunt procedures were done in Canada. Nineteen hundred and seventy-three were shunt insertions and 1,189 were shunt revisions. Based on population, the number of insertions varied between 1 per 5,000 in the province of Nova Scotia to 1 per 20,000 in the province of Manitoba.

The different provinces in Canada keep records of shunting procedures through different health schemes and not all provinces designate the type of shunt inserted. However, of the 1,973 shunts which were inserted during the year 1982/1983, 1,052 were designated as to type. Of this group, 897 or 85.2% were ventriculoperitoneal shunts, 62 or 6.1% were ventriculoatrial shunts, 6 or 0.6% were ventriculocisternostomies or Torkildsen shunts, and 85 or 8.1% were lumboperitoneal shunts.

In the provinces of Quebec and New Brunswick where accurate data are kept with regard to age and sex of patients having shunt insertions, a total of 407 shunts were inserted during the year 1982/1983. Two hundred and sixty-four of these shunts were inserted in males and 213 in females. Two hundred and forty-seven of the patients were children 19 years of age or less and 230 were adults 20 years and older.　　　　　　(Can J Neurol Sci 13: 81–87, 1986)

Key words: Ventriculoperitoneal shunt, Ventriculoatrial shunt, Ventriculocisternostomy, Lumboperitoneal shunt

Summary of CSF Shunt Flow Rates in Eighty Cases

Mitsunori Matsumae, Takeshi Murakami, Toshio Fukuda, Yutaka Suzuki, and Osamu Sato

Departments of Neurosurgery and Nuclear Medicine, Tokai University School of Medicine, Isehara, Kanagawa, Japan

In the report published in the previous year, the authors have pointed out that the flow rate through the CSF shunting system would be greatly influenced by changes in patient's

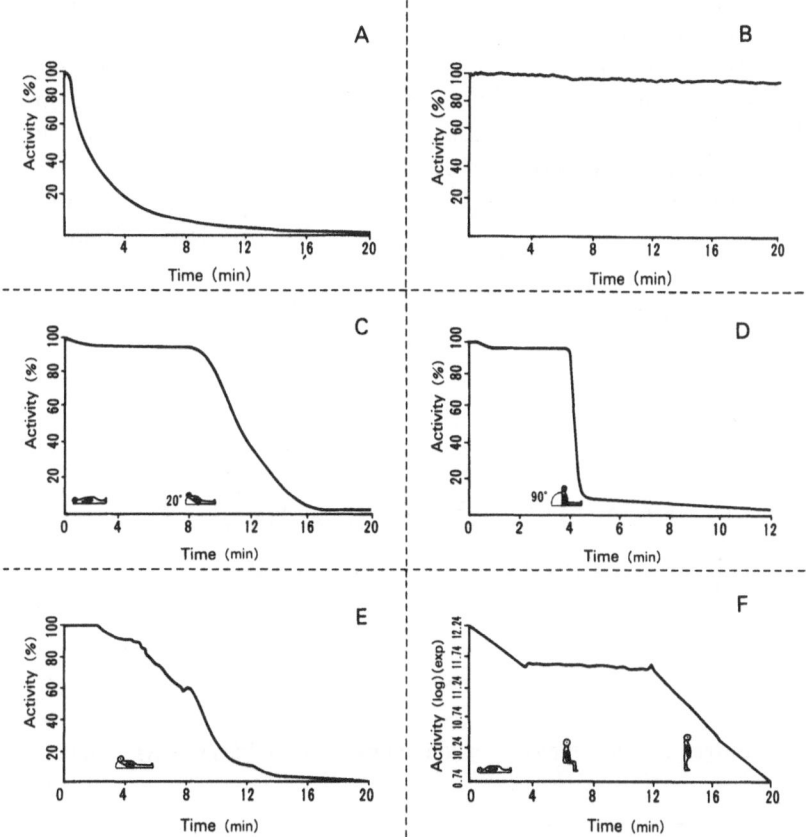

Figure. Measurement of radioactivity. (**A**) The shunt flow rate showed 0.35 ml/min in recumbent position. (**B**) No shunt flow rate in recumbent position. (**C**) The shunt flow rate showed an abrupt increased to 0.25 ml/min in 20 degrees of head raising. (**D**) The shunt flow rate an abrupt increased to 2.5 ml/min in sitting position. (**E**) The shunt flow rate showed increased to 0.10 ml/min at 15 degrees and 0.43 ml/min at 20 degrees. (**F**) The shunt flow rate of 0.36 ml/min in recumbent position become nearly zero in sitting but flow was restored to 0.38 ml/min in upright position.

postures. In this study, we have investigated the effect of the shunting procedures, 80 cases, and the varieties in flow rates as their positional changes being made. Among all the patients studied, 35 cases showed a comparatively satisfactory flow rates of more than 0.11 ml/min in recumbent position, while other 45 cases demonstrated rather slow flow rates of less than 0.10 ml/min in recumbent position. However, even those who such slow flow rates resulted in a favorable prognosis such as flow rate increase on head raising position and eventually decreasing in patient's ventricular size as time passes. To facilitate an early recovery to normal life, it seemed important that the patients should be encouraged to be put in head raising and/or sitting position after the shunt systems are installed. In cases with continuing enlargement of the ventricles and whose flow rates were not increased in head raising, obstruction of the system was suspected. In cases whose flow rates were increased following head raising but who failed to show any reduction in the ventricular size nor clinical improvement, ventriculomegaly due to a severe damage to the cerebral parenchyma were to be considered.

We have already made it clear previously that the flow rate through the shunting system in a patient varies intricately as he changes position in his daily life. Thus far, functions of the shunting system have been assessed by determining the flow rate only in the recumbent position. In the future, however, it will be essential to study the flow rate as postures change. This should lead to a clearer understanding of the circulatory dynamics of the cerebrospinal fluid in shunting system and to proper assessement of the system.

(Annual Report of the Research Committee of "Hydrocephalus," The Ministry of Health and Welfare of Japan, 1986: 127–134, 1987)

Key words: Hydrocephalus, Shunt flow rate, Shunting procedure

An Analysis of Cerebrospinal Fluid Shunt Infections in Adults: A clinical experience of twelve years

Giovanni Spanu

Department of Surgery, Neurosurgical Section, University of Pavia, Pavia, Italy

The authors review their experience on 451 extrathecal CSF shunt in 317 hydrocephalic patients over a period of 12 years. 188 patients were males, 129 females, their age ranged from 13 to 76 years. According to the different shunts patients were subdivided in 4 groups: 114 patients received a ventriculo atrial (VA) shunt, 142 a ventriculo-peritoneal (VP) shunt, 38 an external drainage device and 23 cyst-atrial, cyst-peritoneal or lumbo-peritoneal shunt. In 72 cases (68%) of shunts a revision of the device was necessary due to the obstruction of the ventricular catheter, in 9 cases (8%) the atrial catheter was obstructed; in 10 cases (9%)

of patients who had a VP shunt the peritoneal catheter was obstructed, in other 10 cases (9%) both ventricular and peritoneal catheters were obstructed. In 3 cases the shunt system showed to have a hyperfunction that, in 2 cases, required its demolition.

Thirteen patients of our series are not included in this study because of the existence of a CSF infection prior to surgery.

Our strategy in case of CSF shunt infection was the following: selected antibiotic treatment for 1 weeks; 2 days after the drug suspension patients underwent CSF, blood, urine coltures which were repeated 3 times at a distance of 2 days each. In case of colture negativity patients underwent a new implantation of CSF shunt. Pathogens we found in CSF or shunt coltures were: staphylococcus aureus 11 cases; staphylococcus albus 2 cases; staphylococcus epidermidis 4 cases; enterobacter cloacae 2 cases; serratia marcescens 2 cases; klebsiella pneumoniae 2 cases; hafnia 2 cases; proteus mirabilis, achromobacter species, escherichia coli, pseudomonas aeruginosa, micrococcus and enterococcus 1 case each.

Our opinion is that the main risk factors for infection are: poor skin condition, wrong asepsis procedures and bad air circulation in the operating theatre.

Antibiotic therapy must be chosen according to three criteria: high pathogen sensitivity, proper concentration in ventricular CSF, pharmacocynetics of the drug inside CSF.

According to these selection criteria, in our series, infections decreased from 8% (1972–1978) to 4% (1979–1984).   (Acta Neurochir 80: 79–82, 1986)

Key words: Hydrocephalus, Infections, Cerebrospinal fluid shunt

Table. Aetiology and infections in patients with hydrocephalus

	Aetiology		Infections	
	N° of cases	%	N° of cases	%
Tumour	120	38	11	9
Subarachnoid hemorrhage	95	30	8	8
Head injury	63	20	3	5
Meningitis	13	4	1	8
Miscellaneous	24	8	—	—

Data about aetiology refer to the number of patients (317); data about infections refer to the number of surgical procedure (451).

Staphylococcus Epidermidis Ventriculitis Treated with Vancomycin and Rifampin

Jeffrey S. Osborn, Stanley Sharp, E. Jerome Hanson, Edwin MacGee, and Joseph H. Brewer

Department of Medicine (Infectious Diseases), Medical Education, and Neurosciences, St. Luke's Hospital, Kansas City, Missouri, USA

Cerebrospinal fluid (CSF) shunt infections represent a difficult clinical problem which usually requires removal of the foreign body along with appropriate antimicrobial therapy. Staphylococcus epidermidis is the most common organism isolated from infected CSF shunts. Antimicrobial resistance to S. epidermidis, which may not be reliably predicted by routine laboratory testing, has become an increasingly important problem in the management of these patients. We report two patients with S. epidermidis ventriculitis that persisted on anti-staphylococcal therapy and subsequently responded to Vancomycin and Rifampin.

The first patient was a 9-year-old girl with post-traumatic ventricular hemorrhage requring a ventriculostomy catheter. The catheter became infected with S. epidermidis which persisted despite removal of the foreign body and intravenous (IV) Nafcillin. She subsequently responded to IV Vancomycin, oral Rifampin and intraventricular Vancomycin injections (via a reservoir).

The second patient was an 11-month-old boy with shunt dependent hydrocephalus from birth, who developed S. epidermidis ventriculitis from an infected shunt. The shunt was removed and he was treated with IV Nafcillin. The CSF cultures remained positive. After switching to IV Vancomycin, oral Rifampin and intraventricular Vancomycin, the infection resolved with successful placement of a new shunt.

Although there is limited experience with Vancomycin for CSF infections, the drug represents an important agent for resistant S. epidermidis infections of the CSF. The addition of Rifampin and intraventricular Vancomycin therapy are important adjuncts. Intraventricular Vancomycin appears to be safe and well-tolerated in such patients.

(Neurosurgery 19: 824–827, 1986)

Key words: Rifampin, Shunt infection, Staphylococcus epidermidis, Vancomycin, Ventriculitis

Pharmacokinetics of Intraventricular Vancomycin in Hydrocephalic Rats

Matthew A. Howard,[1] M. Sean Grady,[1] T. S. Park,[1] and W. Michael Scheld[2]

Departments of [1]Neurological Surgery and [2]Internal Medicine, University of Virginia School of Medicine, Charlottesville, Virginia, USA

Patients treated for hydrocephalus are susceptible to developing infectious complications. Ventriculitis is associated with a high mortality and morbidity rate and is often treated with antibiotics administered intraventricularly. Despite the widespread use of intraventricular antibiotics, little is known about the pharmacokinetics of this route of administration in the setting of hydrocephalus.

An inexpensive, reliable animal model of hydrocephalus was developed to investigate the pharmacokinetics of intraventricular vancomycin. Obstructive hydrocephalus was consistently produced in craniectomized adult rats by injecting kaolin into the cisterna magna. After induction of hydrocephalus, 0.05 ml of 0.3 mg/ml vancomycin was injected into the right lateral ventricle of each rat. Bilateral ventricular cerebrospinal fluid (CSF) and brain parenchymal samples were obtained at 0.5, 1, 2, 4, 8 and 12 hours and the concentration of vancomycin in these samples was determined. Brain tissue was also analyzed histologically. The results show: (a) vancomycin is rapidly distributed within the CSF, including the contralateral ventricle, within 30 minutes; (b) vancomycin concentrations were nearly identical in both ventricles at all time points; (c) mean peak CSF vancomycin concentrations occurred at 2 hours and were 23.8 and 21.3 $\mu g/ml$ for the left and right lateral ventricles, respectively; (d) elimination from CSF was slow (T1/2=2.22 hours, T1/2=19.65 hours); (e) no vancomycin was detected (<2 $\mu g/g$) in samples of periventricular white matter; (f) histological changes observed were consistent with untreated obstructive hydrocephalus and did not seem to be related to vancomycin treatment.

The rapid distribution of vancomycin and slow elimination phase lend experimental support to the clinical observation that vancomycin injections once a day often are effective in sterilizing the ventricular system. More accurate quantitative extrapolations to the clinical setting may be possible with a modification of this rat model utilizing a functional shunt and experimental ventriculitis. (Neurosurgery 18: 725–729, 1986)

Key words: Cerebrospinal fluid, Hydrocephalus, Intraventricular antibiotics, Meningitis, Vancomycin, Ventricle

Table. CSF vancomycin concentration (μg/ml) following
intraventricular injection into hydrocephalic rats

Rat ID#	Time interval	Left lateral ventricle		Right lateral ventricle	
1	.5 hr.	23.0		18.4	
2	.5 hr.	5.2	x̄=20.2	5.4	x̄=17.6
3	.5 hr.	45.0	SEM=9.2	38.0	SEM=7.4
4	.5 hr.	7.6		8.4	
5	1.0 hr.	5.3		5.1	
6	1.0 hr.	13.0	x̄=17.6	12.0	x̄=18.0
7	1.0 hr.	21.0	SEM=5.5	20.0	SEM=6.4
8	1.0 hr.	31.0		35.0	
9	2.0 hr.	21.0		23.0	
10	2.0 hr.	24.5	x̄=23.8	19.0	x̄=21.3
11	2.0 hr.	26.0	SEM=1.5	22.0	SEM=1.2
12	4.0 hr.	8.7		8.7	
13	4.0 hr.	12.3		12.4	
14	4.0 hr.	13.5	x̄=10.7	10.7	x̄=11.7
15	4.0 hr.	9.7	SEM=0.9	8.2	SEM=1.9
16	4.0 hr.	9.4		18.5	
17	8.0 hr.	3.7		3.5	
18	8.0 hr.	5.5	x̄=4.5	4.3	x̄=4.4
19	8.0 hr.	4.4	SEM=0.4	4.8	SEM=0.3
20	8.0 hr.	4.3		4.9	
21	12.0 hr.	4.3		4.1	
22	12.0 hr.	4.3	x̄=3.4	≤2.0*	x̄=1.8
23	12.0 hr.	3.8	SEM=0.8	≤2.0*	SEM=0.8
24	12.0 hr.	≤2.0*		≤2.0*	

x̄=Mean value.
SEM=Standard error of the mean.
* When calculating x̄ and SEM for these points a value of 1.0 was
  assigned.

Ventriculoatrial Shunt Infection Due to Cryptococcus Neoformans:
An ultrastructural and quantitative microbiological study

Thomas J. WALSH, Robert SCHLEGEL, Marcia M. MOODY, John W. COSTERTON, and Michael SALCMAN

Division of Infectious Diseases, University of Maryland Cancer Center and Division of Neurosurgery, University of Maryland Hospital, Baltimore, Maryland, USA; and Department of Biology, University of Calgary, Calgary, Canada

The principal cause of infection of ventriculatrial shunts is Staphylococcus epidermis. Fungi have seldom been documented as a cause of infection. Moreover, ultrastructural and quantitative microbiological features of such infections have not been well studied. A 28-year-old man with a ventriculoatrial shunt presented with fever and signs of shunt obstruction in November 1983. The shunt was inserted in 1982 to replace an obstructed shunt inserted for noncommunicating hydrocephalus that was reportedly due to aseptic meningitis as a child. The cerebrospinal fluid (CSF) culture in 1982 was negative for bacteria, fungi, and mycobacteria. The new intraoperative CSF sample grew C.neoformans. CSF white blood cell count was $4/mm^3$ (64% polymorphonuclear leukocytes and 36% lymphocytes), 10 red blood cells/mm^3, protein 45mg/dl, and glucose 6 mg/dl. Cryptococcal antigen titer was 1:32. The ventriculoatrial shunt was removed under sterile conditions and transferred to a sterile transport container. Sections A, B, and C (0.5 cm each) were cut from the catheter, suspended in 10 ml of sterile 0.1 M phosphate-buffered saline (pH 7.0), and shaken in a Vortex mixer for 30 seconds. Serial 10-fold dilutions of the suspension were plated on Sabouraud's dextrose agar and sheep's blood agar plates. Colony counts were read after 48 hours. Adjacent sections of the shunt corresponding to those quantitatively cultured were prepared for scanning electron microscopy. Scanning electron microscopy demonstrated a biofilm and numerous yeasts covering the surface of the ventricular portion of the catheter, consistent with C.neoformans. Yeast-like organisms were rarely seen on the pump portion of the catheter tip. No bacteria were seen within the biofilm or on any portion of the shunt. The ventricular catheter (Section C) demonstrated the highest concentration of C. neoformans, 9×10^6 colony-forming units (CFU)/0.5-cm segment. C.neoformans measured at the junction (Section B) between the ventricular catheter tip and pump was 5×10^4 CFU/0.5-cm segment. The vascular segment grew only 1×10^2 CFU/0.5-cm segment. Thus, a concentration gradient of C. neoformans occurred along the ventriculoatrial shunt with fungi found in highest concentrations on the ventricular catheter and in lowest concentrations at the vascular segment. These findings suggests a ventriculitis or encephalitis as the primary process with extension outward to the meningeal surface. (Neurosurgery 18: 373–375, 1986)

Key words: Cryptococcus neoformans, Hydrocephalus, Shunt infection, Ventriculoatrial shunt

Table. Quantitative microbiology of the ventriculoatrial shunt

Segment designation	Component of shunt	Organism (CFU/0.5 cm)
A	Vascular tip	C. neoformans (1×10^2)
B	Ventricular catheter/pump connection	C. neoformans (5×10^4)
C	Ventricular catheter	C. neoformans (9×10^6)

Spontaneous Intracerebral Pneumocephalus after Ventriculoperitoneal Shunting in Patients with Posterior Fossa Tumors: Report of two cases

Akira Tanaka, Naoki Matsumoto, Takeo Fukushima and Masamichi Tomonaga

Department of Neurosurgery, Fukuoka University, Fukuoka, Japan

A 47-year-old man was admitted with hearing loss of the left ear and blurred vision. There was advanced papilledema. A CT scan demonstrated a round tumor of the left cerebellopontine angle, with associated hydrocephalus. A suboccipital craniectomy was performed, and this acoustic neuroma was totally removed. The operative site developed a pseudomeningocele 1 month later and a ventriculoperitoneal shunt was placed, with subsequent shrinkage of the enlarged ventricles and collapse of the wound bulging. Two weeks later, the patient complained of headache and a bubbling sound. A CT scan disclosed air influx into the ventricles through a porencephalic cavity of the left temporal lobe. A 39-year-old man came to our department with hearing difficulty on the left side and unsteady gait. There was advanced papilledema. A CT scan revealed an enhancing tumor and associated cyst in the left cerebellopontine angle and enlarged ventricles. A ventriculoperitoneal shunt collapsed the ventricles. A suboccipital craniectomy was performed, and a neuroma of the jugular foramen was totally removed. Eight months later, he noticed a bubbling sound in the head. A CT scan demonstrated air in a porencephalic cavity of the left temporal lobe and in the ventricles.

On both cases, a left temporal craniotomy was subsequently done. In each instance, the meningocerebral cicatrix plugged the small defect of the petrous bone in the tegmen tympani through which the mastoid air cells were visualized. The separation of the cicatrized cortex from the dura mater revealed the entrance of the porencephalic cavity of the temporal lobe through which air and CSF could leak. The closure of the dural defect prevented the further inflow of air to the ventricles.

Thinning of the petrous bone may occur secondary to chronic hydrocephalus or congenital factors. The decrease of intracranial pressure after a shunt might play a role in causing pneumocephalus.   (Neurosurgery 18: 499–501, 1986)

Key words: Hydrocephalus, Petrous bone, Pneumocephalus, Ventriculoperitoneal shunt

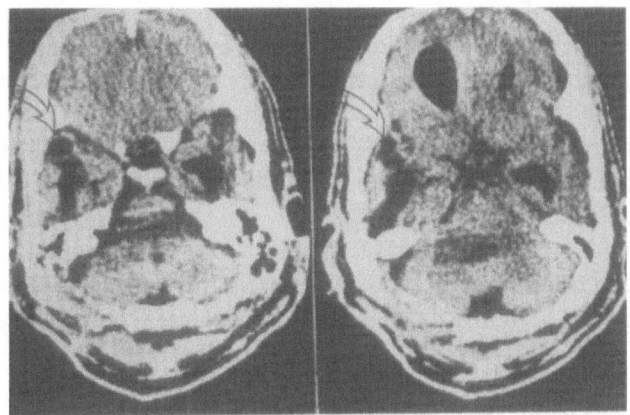

Figure. Case 1. CT scan on second admission shows the air in a porencephalic cavity of the left temporal lobe (*left*) and the air in the ventricle (*right*).

Delayed Intracerebral Hemorrhage after Ventriculoperitoneal Shunting

Robert B. Snow, Robert D. Zimmerman, and Orrin Devinsky

Department of Neurosurgery, Neuroradiology, Neurology, The New York Hospital-Cornell Medical Center, New York, NY, USA

Intracerebral hemorrhage after a ventricular shunting procedure is uncommon. In our series of 900 shunting procedures we have seen 3 moderate sized hemorrhages (3 to 5 cm in size) for an incidence of 0.3%. One of these cases developed the hemorrhage one week after an uneventful ventricular shunting procedure. The patient left the hospital on the 5th postoperative day feeling well. On the 7th postoperative day she developed a headache and had a generalized convulsion. On readmission she was lethargic, with a stiff neck and a mild left hemiparesis. A CT scan and MRI scan revealed a 3–5 cm right frontal intraparenchymal hematoma along the path of the ventricular catheter. A cerebral angiogram was normal. The patient had had no trauma since the shunting procedure. She had no history of bleeding disorder, and hematological tests including platelet count, prothrombin time, partial thromboplastin time, and bleeding time were all within normal limits. The patient fully recovered without operative intervention.

There are several possible mechanisms whereby intracerebral hemorrhage can occur after ventricular shunting procedures: (a) a coexistant bleeding disorder, (b) shunt-induced disseminated intravascular coagulation, (c) disruption of an intracerebral vessel by the catheter, (d) hemorrhage into an intracerebral tumor, (e) hemorrhage from an occult vascular malformation, and (f) head trauma occurring shortly after shunt placement. In the present case the most likely mechanism is disruption of a cerebral blood vessel by the catheter. The normal pulsations of the cerebrospinal fluid transmitted to the ventricular catheter may have caused the catheter to erode through a blood vessel with subsequent intracerebral hemorrhage.

There have been no other reports in the literature documenting delayed intracerebral hemorrhage after a shunting procedure. We present this unusual case to add to the literature list of complications after ventricular shunting procedures. (Neurosurgery 19: 305–307, 1986)

Key words: Intracerebral hemorrhage, Postoperative complication, Ventriculoperitoneal shunt

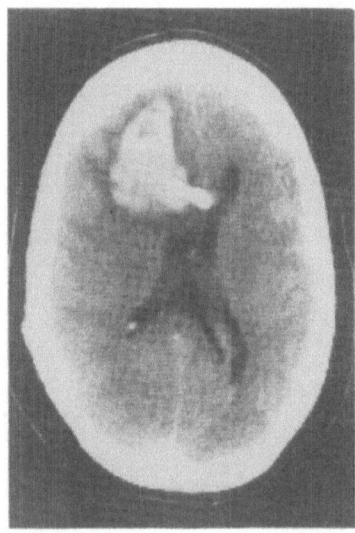

Figure. CT scan without contrast that was obtained on postoperative day 7. A moderate-sized hematoma surrounds the ventricular catheter.

Perimesencephalic Cistern Obliteration:
A CT sign of life-threatening shunt failure

Dennis L. JOHNSON, Charles FITZ, David C. McCULLOUGH, and Saul SCHWARZ

Departments of Neurosurgery and Radiology, Children's Hospital National Medical Center, Washington, D.C.; and Department of Neurosurgery, Bethesda Naval Hospital, Bethesda, Maryland, USA

Although it is rare that a child dies from shunt malfunction, every experienced pediatric neurosurgeon is aware of patients who precipitously deteriorate on the ward while being observed for diagnostic confirmation of their hydrocephalus or while awaiting scheduled surgery. We are presenting eight cases of shunt malfunction who were arousable on admission and scheduled for shunt revision the following day. A precipitous decline in neurologic status prompted unscheduled emergency shunt revision in each case. In fact, six of the eight patients demonstrated decerebrate posturing just prior to surgery. Three patients had a cardiopulmonary arrest and two of the patients died. Most children had been revised several times before but had never undergone urgent surgery. Their clinical histories were not suggestive of extreme shunt dependence. Most of the older children had headaches for five days or more and the majority had been vomiting for more than 24 hours. Furthermore, there were no physical signs that suggested marginal compliance. No patient had papilledema, and only two children had new eye signs. No pupillary changes were manifest. Review of the CT scans revealed ventriculomegaly with previously documented smaller

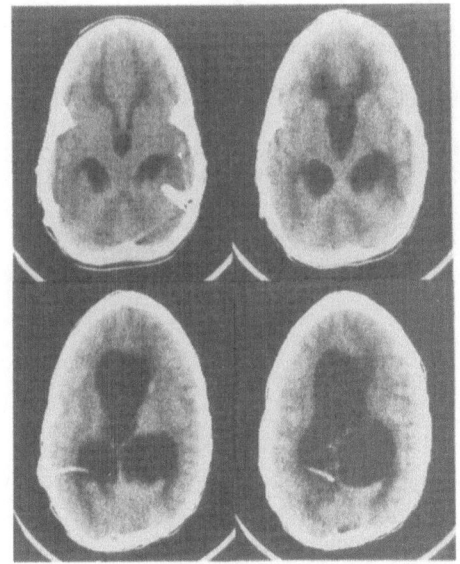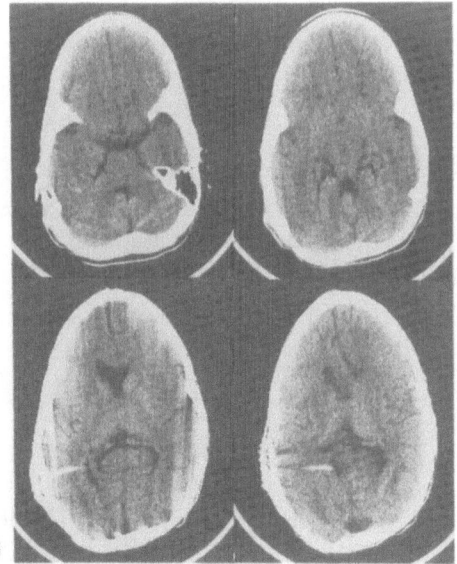

Figure. (A) Shunt failure with perimesencephalic cistern obliteration.
(B) Reappearance of cistern after shunt revision.

ventricles. More importantly, the basilar cisterns were not seen on any preoperative scan, but were visible postoperatively in the survivors. To weigh the importance of this observation, we reviewed the histories and CT scans of 50 cases of hydrocephalus randomly taken from the neuroradiology files at Children's Hospital National Medical Center. Obliteration of the basilar cisterns proved to be a reliable radiographic sign of shunt malfunction requiring emergent attention.   (J Neurosurg 64: 386–389, 1986)

Key words: Basilar cisterns, Shunt failure, Ventriculoperitoneal shunt

Reaction of Rabbit Lateral Periventricular Tissue to Shunt Tubing Implants

Marc R. Del Bigio and J. Edward Bruni

Department of Anatomy, The University of Manitoba, Winnipeg, Canada

The reaction of the periventricular tissue of the lateral ventricle to silicone rubber shunt tubing was studied by light and scanning and transmission electron microscopy. Non-functioning shunt tubing was implanted into the frontal horns of the lateral ventricles of

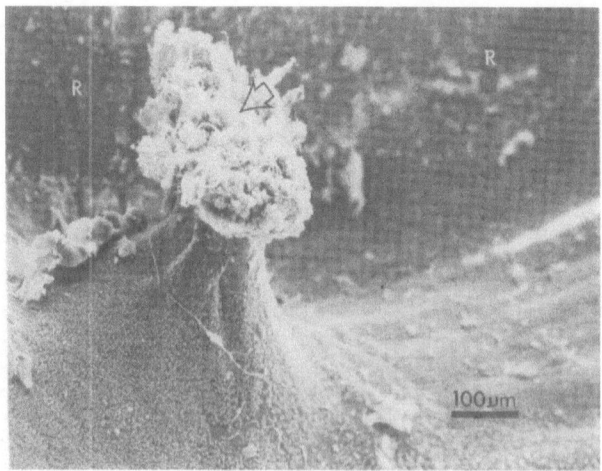

Figure. Scanning electron micrograph showing a ventricular wall outgrowth at three weeks post-implantation. The outgrowth is partially covered by ependyma at the base but astroglial cells and processes are exposed to the ventricle at the apex (*arrow*). R=roof of the lateral ventricle.

rabbits which were then sacrificed at intervals of 3 days to 16 weeks thereafter. Colchicine was used to study mitotic activity in the region of the shunt. Reactive changes that occurred in the periventricular tissue correlated with the degree of contact with the implant and with the duration of the implant period. Ependymal cells underwent progressive attenuation and sloughed completely in the most severely affected areas. Prominent gliosis in the subependymal region accompanied the ependymal changes. The ventricular surface directly adjacent to the holes in the implant developed ependymal covered glial evaginations which grew into the implant holes beginning at one week post-implantation. In the region of the outgrowths, ependymal mitotic activity was significantly increased at one and two weeks post-implantation and astroglial mitotic activity was increased at three days and one week. Proliferation of ependymal and glial cells in the area touching the shunt tubing along with mechanical factors contributed to the development of cellular outgrowths that may be a factor in the pathogenesis of shunt obstruction in human hydrocephalus.

(J Neurosurg 64: 932–940, 1986)

Key words: Astroglia, Cerebral ventricle, Ependyma, Shunt, Silicone

Eosinophilia in the Cerebrospinal Fluid of Children with Shunts Implanted for the Treatment of Internal Hydrocephalus

Elena M. Tzvetanova and Christo T. Tzekov

Institute of Neurology, Psychiatry and Neurosurgery, Medical Academy, Sofia, Bulgaria

The silicon rubber used for the production of shunts in surgical treatment of internal hydrocephalus is tolerated by the patients. Nevertheless, changes in the cell count of CSF including eosinophilia have been reported after shunt implication. We investigated 615 ventricle and 35 lumbar fluids collected from 404 children after the implantation of shunts for cell count, total protein, albumin, glucose, IgG, IgA and chloride levels. Eosinophilia was found in the CSF of 26 (6.4%). Eosinophilic granulocytes constituting 1 to 3% of the cell population were found in 24 cases with an excess of 4% observed only in two cases (0.5%) as a complication of shunt implantation.

In 10 of the 24 children, the same level of eosinophilia was found previous to the shunt operation. Blood eosinophilia was not present in the 26 patients with CSF eosinophilia. Case 1 with extremely high CSF eosinophilia was a three-month-old child to whom shunt was inserted (*Table*) and after that removed due to signs indicative of meningoencephalitis. Case 2 (*Table*) was also three-month-old child with extremely high CSF eosinophilia to whom cyst-atrial shunts was created. Frank CSF eosinophilia is usually observed in parasitic infections of CNS and in some inflammatory dissorders. The introduction of the silicon rubber shunt in neurosurgery has resulted in a new, though infrequent cause of CSF pleocytosis *i.e.* eosinophilia. In patients with hydrocephalia but without shunts up to 5% eosinophilia have been found in isolated cases. Our data show that children with internal hydrocephalus with or without shunts, may have various CSF changes—elevated protein levels, mild leucocytosis involving lymphocytes, and monocytes as well as slight neutrophilic and eosinophilic reaction. Some characteristic findings in the two cases cited are worth mentioning. CSF pleocytosis after shunt was very high as in bacterial meningitis, although the micro biologic tests were negative. Eosinophilia was isolated only in the CSF and was absent in the peripheral blood. Hence, we conclude that the allergic reaction of the ependyma remained localized within the CNS. No doubt the changes of other CSF parameters resulted from circulatory disturbances of the permeability of the blood-CSF barrier.   (Acta Cytol 30: 277–280, 1986)

Key words: Eosinophilia, Hydrocephalia, Cerebrospinal fluid, Shunt

Table. CSF findings in Cases 1 and 2 with eosinophilia

Date of investig	Leu /1	Eo %	Neu %	Ly %	Mo %	M° %	T.Pr g/l	Alb g/l	IgG mg/l	IgA mg/l	Glu mmol/l	Chlor mmol/l	Blood Eo %
Case 1													
10/14/83	8	0	2	65	30	3	6.9	—	60	11	1.4	112	3
11/4/83 (shunt implanted)	9	0	0	67	31	2	3.7	—	—	—	1.1	113	2
11/15/83 (shunt removed)	1,746	68	3	23	6	0	6.4	4.2	72	16	1.8	115	4
11/29/83	68	53	8	22	14	3	1.7	3.1	43	9	2.0	123	4
12/5/83	66	3	1	54	35	7	1.7	—	—	—	2.2	122	3
1/5/84	10	1	0	65	34	0	1.0	0.7	38	8	2.2	118	3
1/12/84	6	0	2	66	32	0	1.13	—	—	—	2.3	119	—
1/19/84	11	0	0	74	25	1	0.8	—	—	—	2.4	118	3
Case 2													
12/15/84	3	0	4	54	40	2	0.1	0.04	—	—	3.3	119	4
3/20/84 (shunt implanted)	7	0	5	55	39	1	0.15	0.04	16	3	3.4	117	4
5/20/84	8	10	34	45	11	0	0.3	—	—	—	3.4	118	5
6/11/84	171	50	7	35	8	0	1.56	0.85	34	7	2.0	118	5
6/12/84	320	43	6	19	25	7	1.11	0.72	—	—	1.9	124	4
6/15/84	61	78	4	13	4	1	0.78	0.41	22	5	3.1	120	3
6/19/84	19	60	6	16	14	4	0.57	—	—	—	3.0	117	4
6/25/84	18	49	14	20	15	2	0.42	0.26	17	2	2.7	118	5

Reaction of Periventricular Tissue in the Rat Fourth Ventricle to Chronically Placed Shunt Tubing Implants

J. E. BRUNI and M. R. DEL BIGIO

Department of Anatomy, The University of Manitoba, Winnipeg, Manitoba, USA

The reaction of periventricular tissue to shunt tubing chronically implanted in the fourth ventricle of the rat was investigated by correlative scanning and transmission electron microscopy. Sterile silicone tubing with four 0.4 mm diameter holes was inserted into the fourth ventricle of adult Sprague-Dawley rats through an incision in the atlanto-occipital membrane and the animals were killed at post-operative intervals of 5 and 8 weeks. Reactive changes that could be correlated with the extent of contact with the implant occurred in the periventricular tissue. The ependyma lining the ventricle underwent a progressive loss of cilia and microvilli, became attenuated and, in circumscribed areas, was lost entirely. A significant subependymal gliosis accompanied these changes. In regions denuded of ependyma, neurons and glia were exposed directly to the cerebrospinal fluid. Eruptions of periventricular tissue corresponding precisely to the location of holes in the implanted tubing were observed on both the vermal surface of the cerebellum and the floor of the ventricle. Evaginations from the surface of the inferior vermis and the floor of the ventricle were most prevalent at 5 and greatest at 8 weeks post-implantation, respectively. Gliosis combined with mechanical factors are believed to be responsible for development of these periventricular

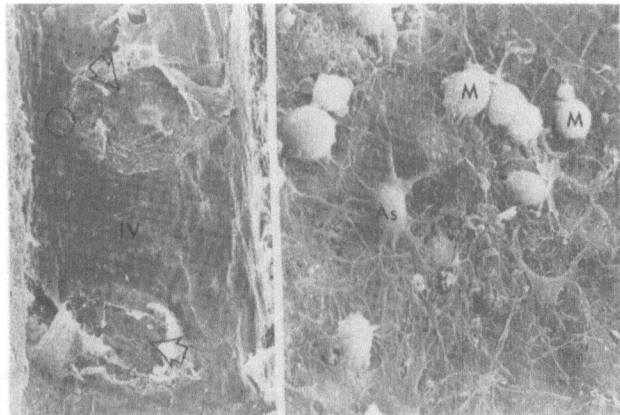

Figure. *Left*, Floor of the rat fourth ventricle (IV) 5 weeks postimplantation showing two evaginations (*arrows*) corresponding to the location of holes in the silicone tubing. ×100. *Right*, enlargement of an area of ependymal erosion on a tissue eruption comparable to that encircled in the figure on the left. Numerous stellate cells presumed to be glial (As) and a complex meshwork of processes have been exposed to the CSF. (M), macrophages; 5 weeks post-implantation. ×3560.

tissue evaginations, which may be a factor in the pathogenesis of cerebrospinal fluid shunt obstruction in treated human hydrocephalus.   (Neurosurgery 19: 337–345, 1986)

Key words: Cytopathology, Electron microscopy, Fourth ventricle, Rat, Shunt

Large Extra-abdominal Cyst as a Postpartum Complication of Peritoneal Shunt: Case report

Philip NUGENT and Sylvio HOSHEK

Departments of General Surgery and Neurosurgery, Kaiser Permanente Medical Center, Los Angles, California, USA

An extra-abdominal cyst filled with cerebrospinal fluid was found postpartum in a patient with a ventriculoperitoneal (VP) shunt. No similar complication of VP shunting has been reported before.

Case Report

This 30-year-old Mexican-American woman was 7 weeks pregnant when she presented in the emergency room with nausea and severe headaches. She was noted to have a depressed sensorium, and an emergency computerized tomography (CT) scan of the head revealed moderate hydrocephalus. She underwent implantation of a right VP shunt with resolution of symptoms. Laboratory studies showed positive titers in the CSF for cysticercosis. The patient had a normal spontaneous vaginal delivery of a healthy baby girl 7 months later. She noticed a slowly enlarging mass 3 weeks postpartum over her abdominal incision, which was soft and not tender. There were no headaches or disturbance of sensorium.

Examination. Physical examination revealed a thin woman in no distress. She had a patent valve in her VP shunt. Abdominal examination revealed normal bowel sounds. She had a 15×10 cm mass over the abdominal incision in her right upper quadrant which was nonreducible. Admission laboratory studies were unremarkable.

Operation. The old incision was opened and a 15×10-cm cyst was found completely extraperitoneally with the intraperitoneal portion of the VP shunt coiled inside it. The peritoneal portion of the catheter was replaced and implanted correctly into the abdominal cavity.

Postoperative Course. The patient left the hospital on the 3rd postoperative day. She has been followed for 23 months and is free of symptoms. The shunt is functioning well.

(J Neurosurg 64: 151–152, 1986)

Key words: Cyst, Ventriculoperitoneal shunt, Abdominal wall cyst, Postpartum complica-
                tion

Liver Abscess Following Penetration of the Liver with a Ventriculo-Peritoneal Shunt Tube: An unusual complication of a ventriculo-peritoneal shunt

Shozo Yamada,[1] Tadashi Aiba,[1] Shozi Yoshiwara,[2] and Kunihiko Akagi[2]

Departments of [1]Neurosurgery and [2]Pediatrics, Toranomon Hospital, Tokyo, Japan

Liver abscess complicating ventriculo-peritoneal shunt as a result of penetration of the liver by the abdominal shunt catheter is extremely rare. To our knowledge, only one case has so far been reported in the literature.

A five-year-old boy with choroid-plexus papilloma and hydrocephalus was treated by routine ventriculo-peritoneal shunt. The Pudentz shunt system was used with the distal catheter positioned in the supra-hepatic cavity. Two years eight months later, he was re-admitted to our hospital because of pyrexia (39.5°C) and leucocytosis. Ten days prior to re-admission, he was held by his feet and swung around during play in his kindergarden. Since then he developed malaise followed by pyrexia. The diagnosis of liver abscess secondary to the penetration of liver by shunt catheter was established by means of abdominal ultrasonography and computed axial tomography (*Figure*). The patient was managed by shunt externalization and appropriate antibiotics. Pseudomonas multophilia was isolated from the peritoneal catheter. In this patient, it might be possible that the rather "sharp" distal tip of the Pudentz catheter in the suprahepatic cavity could have penetrated the liver when the child was swung around during play. Liver abscess subsequently developed around the tip of the penetrated catheter. In conclusion, the authors emphasized the value of abdominal ultrasonography and especially computed axial tomography which can provide a definitive diagnosis of this disease entity and should be considered for patients who developed

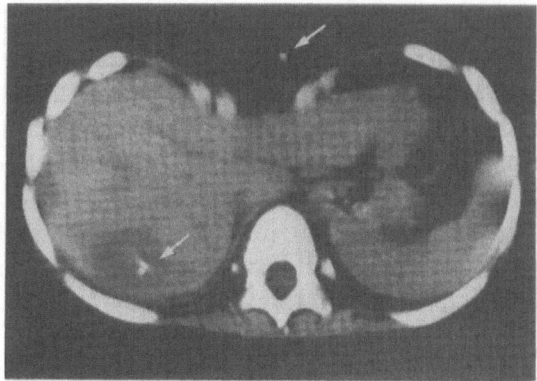

Figure. CT scan at the level of the liver shows an ill-defined, rounded, low density abscess in the right lobe of the liver. Shunt tube is seen both subcutaneously and within the abscess (*arrow*).

abdominal symptoms and signs with pyrexia of unknown origin following ventriculo-
peritoneal shunt.   (*Shoni no Noshinkei* 11: 39–44, 1986)

Key words: Ventriculo-peritoneal shunt, Abdominal complication, Penetration of the liver,
Liver abscess, Pseudomonas maltophilia

The Incidence of Epilepsy after Ventricular Shunting Procedures

Noel G. Dan and Megan J. Wade

Departments of Neurosurgery and Medical Records, Concord Hospital, Sydney, New South Wales,
Australia

Two hundred seven consecutive patients with ventricular shunts were studied. 27 were
excluded because seizures had occurred before shunting. 17 of the remaining 180 patients
(9.4%) developed seizures. Follow-up was a minimum of two years unless death occurred
during the second year. Prophylactic anticonvulsant drugs were not used routinely. 5/21 of
those on anticonvulsants developed seizures, despite the anticonvulsants. No pattern related
to the underlying disorder was apparent amongst the 17 patients who developed epilepsy.
There was a clear gradation related to age falling from 15.2% in those under one year to
6.9% in those over fifty years. This was not of statistical significance ($P=0.1$).
No convulsions occurred during the first 14 days after shunting but 52.9% occurred within
one year and 76.4% within two years of shunt placement. In the third year there was a 1%
risk of developing epilepsy and a 1% risk remained thereafter.
As cortical trauma was suspected to be the most important factor in the development of
epilepsy, cortical penetration was studied. No difference was found between unilateral and
bilateral ventricular catheterizations. Frequency of revision had a significant relationship to
the occurrence of seizures being 5.9% in those without revisions increasing to over 20% in
those with two or three shunt revisions ($P=0.05$).
The anatomical site of cortical puncture revealed a significant difference in incidence
($P=0.01$). Ten of 168 patients (6.6%) with a posterior parietal puncture suffered seizures. Six
of eleven with a frontal catheterization (54.5%) became epileptic. All six, however, did
experience shunt revisions.
Whilst the overall 9.4% incidence of epilepsy after shunting is lower than other recorded
series, it remains a significant incidence. Further investigation appears indicated.
                                                      (J Neurosurg 65: 19–21, 1986)

Key words: Ventricular shunt, Epilepsy, Hydrocephalus, Cerebrospinal fluid diversion

Table. Time to onset of ictus after ventricular shunting in 17 seizure patients

Time	No. of Cases	Percent of Seizure Cases	Percent of Total Series
0–14 days	0	0	0
2–8 wks	6	35.3	3.3
9–52 wks	3	17.6	1.7
1–2 yrs	4	23.5	2.2
2–3 yrs	2	11.8	1.1
>3 yrs	2	11.8	1.1
total cases	17	100	9.4

Slit Like Ventricle and Isolation of the CSF Pathway as Complications of Shunt Procedure in Child Hydrocephalus: (Part-6) Pathophysiology and treatment of isolated unilateral hydrocephalus

Shizuo Oi[1] and Satoshi Matsumoto[2]

[1]Department of Neurosurgery, National Kagawa Children's Hospital, Zentsuji; and [2]Department of Neurosurgery, Kobe Univrsity School of Medicine, Kobe, Japan

Isolated unilateral hydrocephalus was defined as;

i) Shunt complication which occurred in an initially bilaterally expanded communicating lateral ventricle.

ii) Reexpansion of the contralateral ventricle after a unilateral shunt placemant.

iii) Progressive hydrocephalus with no evidence of a primary destructive lesion, *e.g.* porencephaly.

The treatment and prevention were discussed on the basis of critical analysis of the pathophysiology.

All of the cases were shunted in the neonatal period or early infancy. The symptoms of isolated unilateral hydrocephalus appeared as unilateral cranial expansion with or without contralateral hemiparesis were nystagmus, conjugate deviation or other eye symptoms. The follow-up CT's demonstrated the progressively reexpanding contralateral lateral ventricle while the shunted side became slit-like with the overdraining well-functioning shunt in place.

Analysis of the CSF dynamics by metrizamide or pneumoventriculography/cisternography suggested the existence of a one-way ball valve action of the Foramen of Monro.

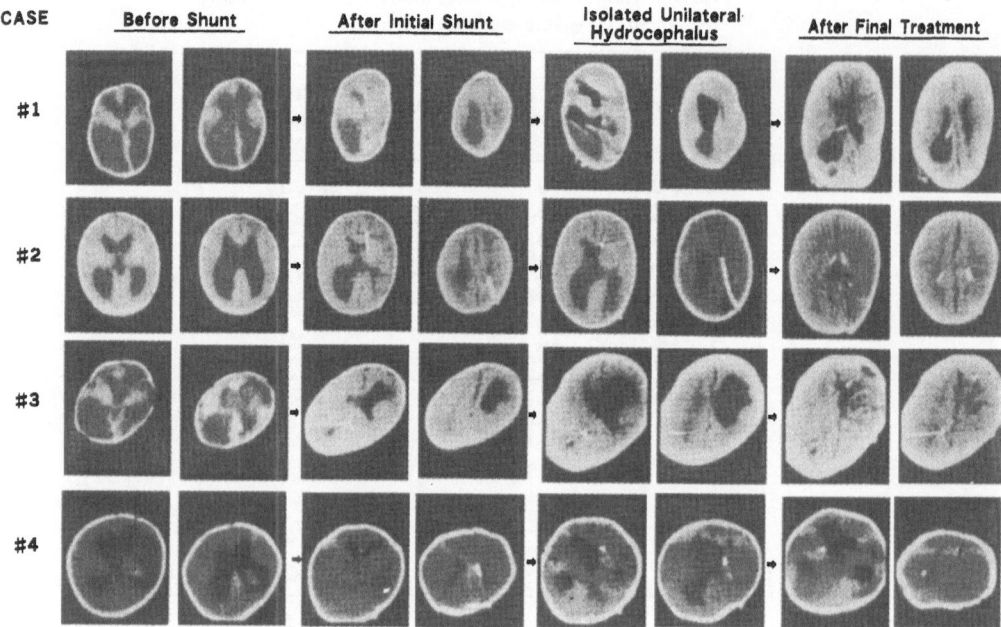

Figure. CT findings of postshunt isolated unilateral hydrocephalus.

Table. Summary of and concepts in isolated unilateral hydrocephalus

---

Definition
- Shunt complication occurred in initially bilaterally expanded communicating lateral ventricle.
- Reexpansion of contralateral ventricle after unilateral shunt placement.
- Progressive hydrocephalus and no evidence of primary destructive lesion e.g. porencephaly.

Causative factors
- Overdrainage of CSF with rapid alteration of bilateral intraventricular pressure balance.
- Underlying inflammatory reaction.
- Immature young brain with high compliance.

Pathophysiology
- CAF Dynamics: Obstructed foramen of Monro, either functional or morphological.
- ICP Dynamics: Independent bilateral intraventricular pressure pattern.

Symptomatology
- Unilateral cranial expansion.
- Unilateral pyramidal tract signs with or without other long tract signs.
- Unilateral visual symptoms e.g. hemianopsia, nystagmus, conjugate deviation.

Treatment
- Flow control of overdraining initial shunt.
- Upgrading pressure of overdraining initial shunt.
- Bilateral shunting with a contralateral additional shunt.

Continuous and simultaneous bilateral intraventricular pressure monitoring on their pulse pressure and compliance revealed independent patterns with pressure gradient.

The pathophysiology of isolated unilateral hydrocephalus demonstrated in this study can be classified into the following two categories:

i) Permanent isolated unilateral hydrocephalus,

ii) Reversible isolated unilateral hydrocephalus.

The treatment should be based on the pathophysiology of occlusion of the Foramen of Monro. (*Shoni no Noshinkei* 11 : 249–256, 1986)

Key words: Hydrocephalus, Shunt complication, Isolated ventricle, Slit-like ventricle, Hydrodynamics, Intraventricular pressure

A Case of Isolated Fourth Ventricle Due to Ruptured Cerebral Aneurysm

Mineko MURAKAMI, Akira TAKAHASHI, Toshiharu MURAKAMI, Hideo ENDO, Iwao SAIKI, and Haruyuki KANAYA

Department of Neurosurgery, Iwate Medical University School of Medicine, Morioka, Japan

We present a case of an isolated fourth ventricle which developed after massive ventricular hemorrhage, due to a ruptured cerebral aneurysm. In an adult, an isolated fourth ventricle seems to be very rare. In addition, the symptoms of unconsciousness and respiratory arrest, as well as the rapid development in this case seemed very unusual. The aqueductal occlusion was considered to be related to the intraventricular hematoma which was still present even at 2 months post-hemorrhage.

This case was a 57-year-old woman admitted to our hospital in a state of coma. CT showed a massive ventricular hematoma and the right carotid angiogram showed an aneurysm of the anterior communicating artery. Bilateral ventricular drainage was performed because of progressive decerebrate rigidity. Since consciousness gradually rose to the Japan Coma Scale 3, clipping of the neck of the aneurysm was performed 25 days after onset. Premature rupture occurred during the operation. After the surgery, CT showed ring-like high densities in both lateral ventricles and also in the fourth ventricle due to the premature rupture of aneurysm. Although the lateral ventricle drainage functioned effectively, the fourth ventricle showed remarkable gradual dilatation. The patient was stuporous, and respiratory arrest occurred suddenly 43 days after onset. Since it was considered that the intraventricular hematoma blocked the aqueduct as well as the outlet of the fourth ventricle, and that the dilated fourth ventricle was compressing the brain stem, a ventriculostomy was performed through a suboccipital craniectomy. The cerebellar hemispheres showed remarkable swelling bilaterally, and no cerebrospinal fluid was found in the cisterna magna. The foramina of Magendie was completely blocked by an old hematoma. When an incision was made in the vermis and the fourth ventricle was opened, red-wine-colored fluid spurted out. After the second surgery, CT showed a decrease in size of the fourth ventricle and the patient's condition improved, due to normal respiration and an improved state of consciousness.

(Noshinkeigeka 14: 817–821, 1986)

Key words: Isolated fourth ventricle, Fourth ventriculostomy, Ruptured aneurysm, Intraventricular hemorrhage

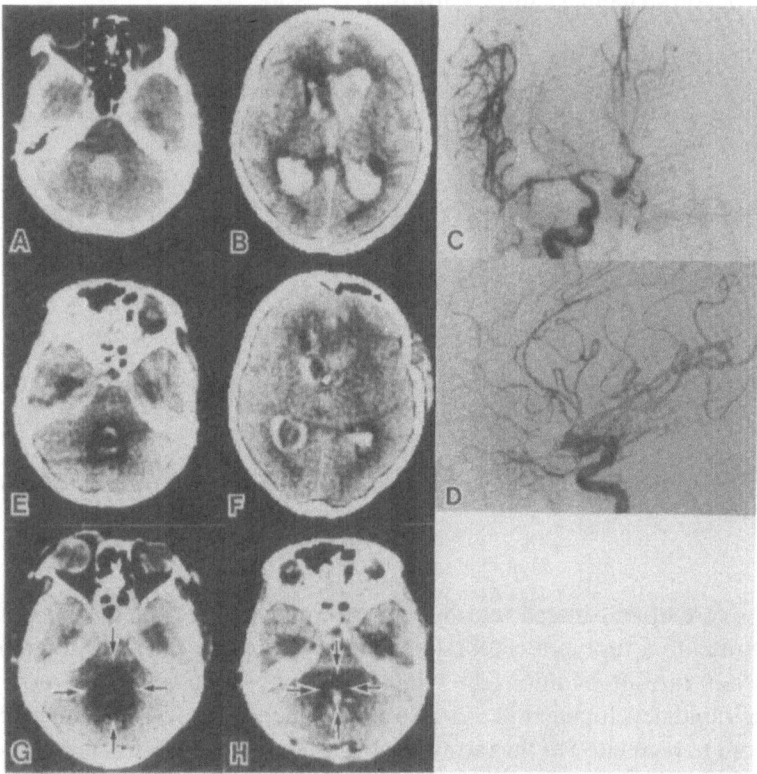

Figure. On admission, CT shows massive ventricular hemorrhage (**A, B**) and right side carotid angiogram reveals an aneurysm of the anterior communicating artery (**C, D**). After the neck clipping of aneurysm, ring-like high densities due to premature rupture of aneurysm are found in lateral and fourth ventricles (**E, F**).

Two days before the second surgery, the fourth ventricle is dilated remarkably (**G**). After ventriculostomy, the fourth ventricle is significantly decreased in size (**H**). The outline of the fourth ventricle is indicated by arrows in Fig. G and H.

Slit Like Ventricle and Isolation of the CSF Pathway as Complications of Shunt Procedure in Childhood Hydrocephalus: (Part-5) Pathogenesis of isolated fourth ventricle

Shizuo Oi[1] and Satoshi Matsumoto[2]

[1]Department of Neurosurgery, National Kagawa Children's Hospital, Zentsuji; and [2]Department of Neurosurgery, Kobe University School of Medicine, Kobe, Japan

The experience with eight cases with an isolated fourth ventricle as a complication of shunt procedures was analyzed and the possible pathogenesis was discussed on the basis of intracranial pressure and hydrodynamic studies.

Symptomatic isolation of the fourth ventricle appeared in seven cases with as long an interval as 6 years and 7 months in average after the initial shunt. Changes in CT findings before the development of the symptomatic isolated fourth ventricle was reviewed and a close relationship between the shunt function and isolation of the fourth ventricle was recognized. The symptoms appeared when the lateral ventricles became slit-like due to overdrainage of cerebrospinal fluid. Change in the size of the lateral ventricles and evident reopening of the aqueductal "functional obstruction" were observed in one case.

Although the pathogenesis of isolated fourth ventricle, especially of secondary aqueductal obstruction, remains unclear, this study strongly suggested that there are two different mechanisms in completion of the isolation of the fourth ventricle. One is "functional obstruction," which is created by shunt overfunction in the lateral ventricle resulted in supratentorial low intraventricular pressure, pulse pressure and compliance. The other one is "morphological obstruction" of the aqueduct, which is the consequence of an inflammatory reaction, peri-aqueductal edema, gliosis and other secondary factors with or without the influence of the shunt procedure.

The choice of the method of treatment for isolated fourth ventricle should be based on the pathophysiology of the mechanism of isolation and varies in cases including veil excision, aqueductal canalization, fourth ventricle shunt, reopening of the associated slit-like ventricle of the lateral ventricles, and others. (*Shoni no Noshinkei* 11: 239–247, 1986)

Key words: Hydrocephalus, Isolated fourth ventricle, Shunt complication, Slit like ventricle

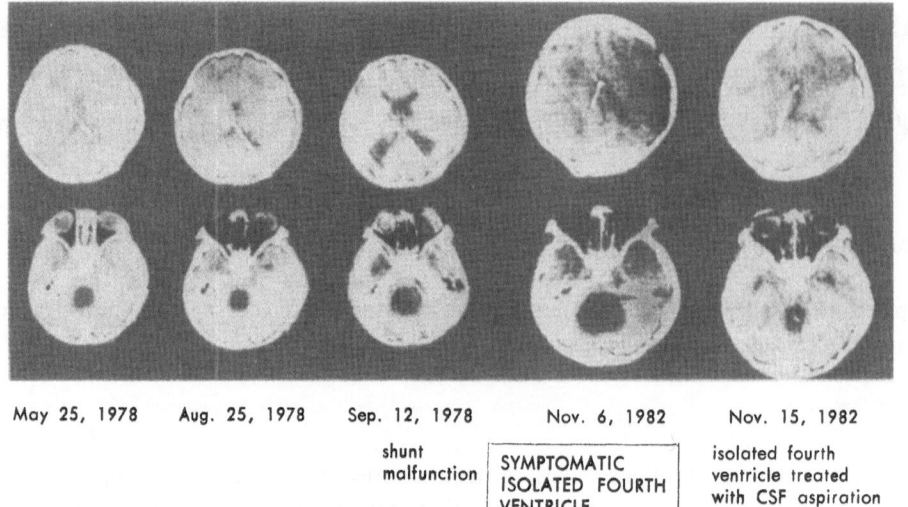

May 25, 1978   Aug. 25, 1978   Sep. 12, 1978   Nov. 6, 1982   Nov. 15, 1982

shunt
malfunction   SYMPTOMATIC
ISOLATED FOURTH
VENTRICLE   isolated fourth
ventricle treated
with CSF aspiration
via Ommaya reservoir

········ASYMPTOMATIC ISOLATED FOURTH VENTRICLE······

Figure. Change of CT findings before development of symptomatic isolated fourth ventricle. Note the relationship between the shunt function and isolation of the fourth ventricle. Symptoms appeared when the lateral ventricles became slit-like.

Table. Treatments and the outcome of symptomatic isolated fourth ventricle. All outcomes were excellent by fourth ventricle-peritoneal shunt in three, intermittent cerebrospinal fluid aspiration in two and opening of the fourth ventricle in one case, respectively as the final treatment

Case	Treatment	Outcomes
1 (K.M.)	• fourth ventricle opening • fourth ventricle-cisterna magna } → • aspiration of CSF via Ommaya reservoir • Placement of antisiphon valve	excellent
2 (C.K.)	• fourth ventricle opening→ • fourth ventricle-peritoneal shunt	excellent
3 (S.M.)	• fourth ventricle-peritoneal shunt	excellent
4 (M.N.)	• aspiration of CSF via Ommaya reservoir	excellent
5 (K.I.)	None	asymptomatic
6 (M.Y.)	None	spontaneously recovered
7 (T.S.)	• aspiration of CSF via Ommaya reservoir → • fourth ventricle-peritoneal shunt	excellent
8 (R.N.)	• fourth ventricle-peritoneal shunt → • fourth ventricle opening	excellent

Pathophysiology of Aqueductal Obstruction in Isolated IV Ventricle after Shunting

Shizuo Oi and Satoshi Matsumoto

Department of Neurosurgery, National Kagawa Children's Hospital, Zentsuji; and Department of Neurological Surgery, Kobe University, School of Medicine, Kobe, Japan

The authors report their cases of isolated IV ventricle and discuss their concepts of secondary obstruction of the aqueduct, analyzing CSF dynamics, pressure measurements, serial CT scan changes, and the outcome of various treatment modalities. Two distinctly different categories were identified: (1) functional obstruction in which the obstructed aqueduct reopened either as the result of decreasing the elevated infratentorial pressure (Raimondi's phenomenon) or from correction of overdrainage of the supratentorial system; (2) permanent obstruction with pathological occlusion of the aqueduct, necessitating a IV ventriculoperitoneal shunt. It is the pathophysiology and pathoanatomy of secondary obstruction of the aqueduct that determine the specific treatment to be used in managing the isolated IV ventricle syndrome.   (Child's Nerv Syst 2: 282–286, 1986)

Key words: Isolated IV ventricle, Hydrocephalus, Shunt complication, CSF dynamics

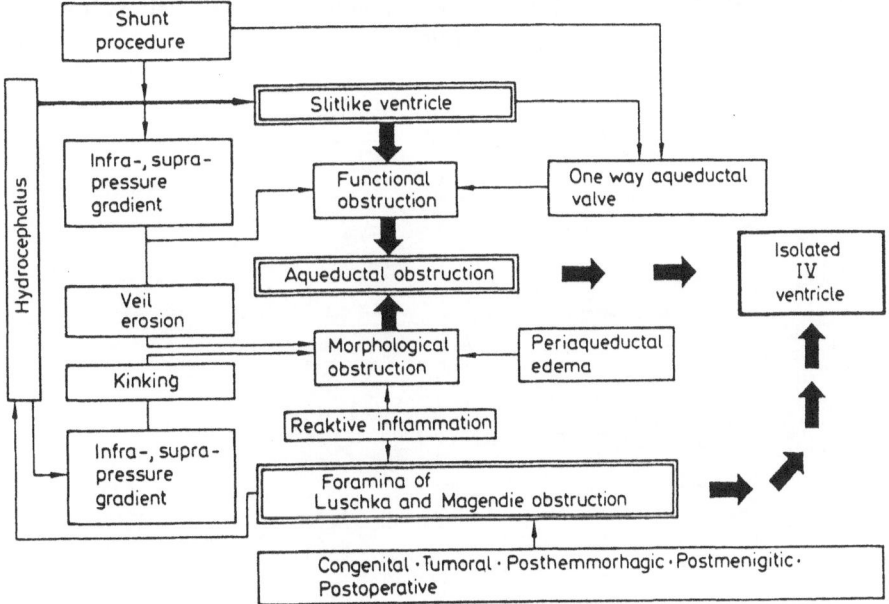

Figure. Possible pathophysiology of postshunt isolated IV ventricle.

Isolated Fourth Ventricle

Shizuo Oi and Satoshi Matsumoto

Department of Neurosurgery, Kobe University, Kobe, Japan

It is now a widely accepted fact that over-drainage of cerebrospinal fluid (CSF) via a CSF shunt could be a causative factor in certain hurmful and occasionally life-threatening conditions, such as the slit ventricle syndrome and isolated CSF pathway.

These clinical entities are recognized as the third most common complication of shunt procedures following shunt malfunction and infection.

The condition of "isolated fourth ventricle" could be defined as follows:

1. CSF shunt complication occurring in hydrocephalus with an initially patent aqueduct.

2. Expansion or reexpansion of the fourth ventricle after CSF shunt placement into the lateral cerebral ventricle.

3. Aqueductal occlusion as a result of CSF overdrainage.

4. Occlusion of the foramina of Magendie and Luschka, probably due to an inflammatory condition associated with the hydrocephalus.

This paper describes the pathophysiology and treatment of isolated fourth ventricle as a form of shunt complication resulting from overdrainage of CSF by an overfunctioning shunt.

(Riv Neurosc Ped (J Ped Neurosc) 2: 125–133, 1986)

Key words: CSF shunt complications, Hydrocephalus, Isolated CSF pathway, Pressure gradient, Aqueductal obstruction

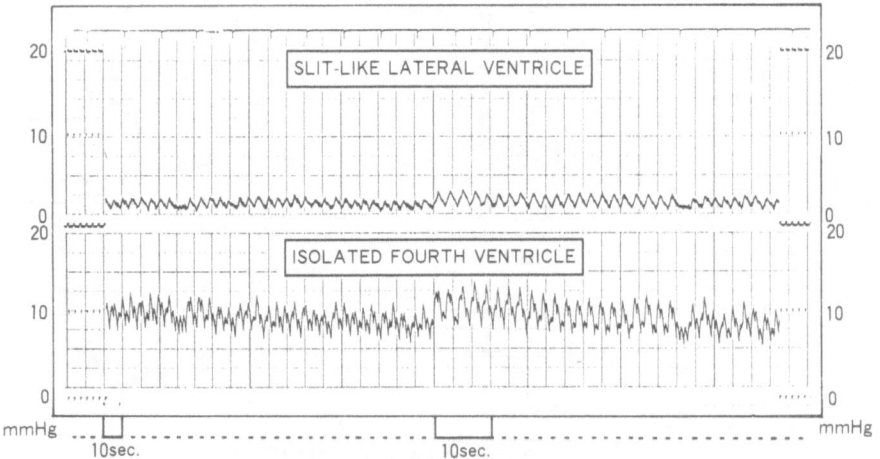

Figure 1. Simultaneous intracranial pressure monitoring from the lateral and fourth ventricles in a case of isolated fourth ventricle. Note the differences between the baseline pressure and pulse pressure.

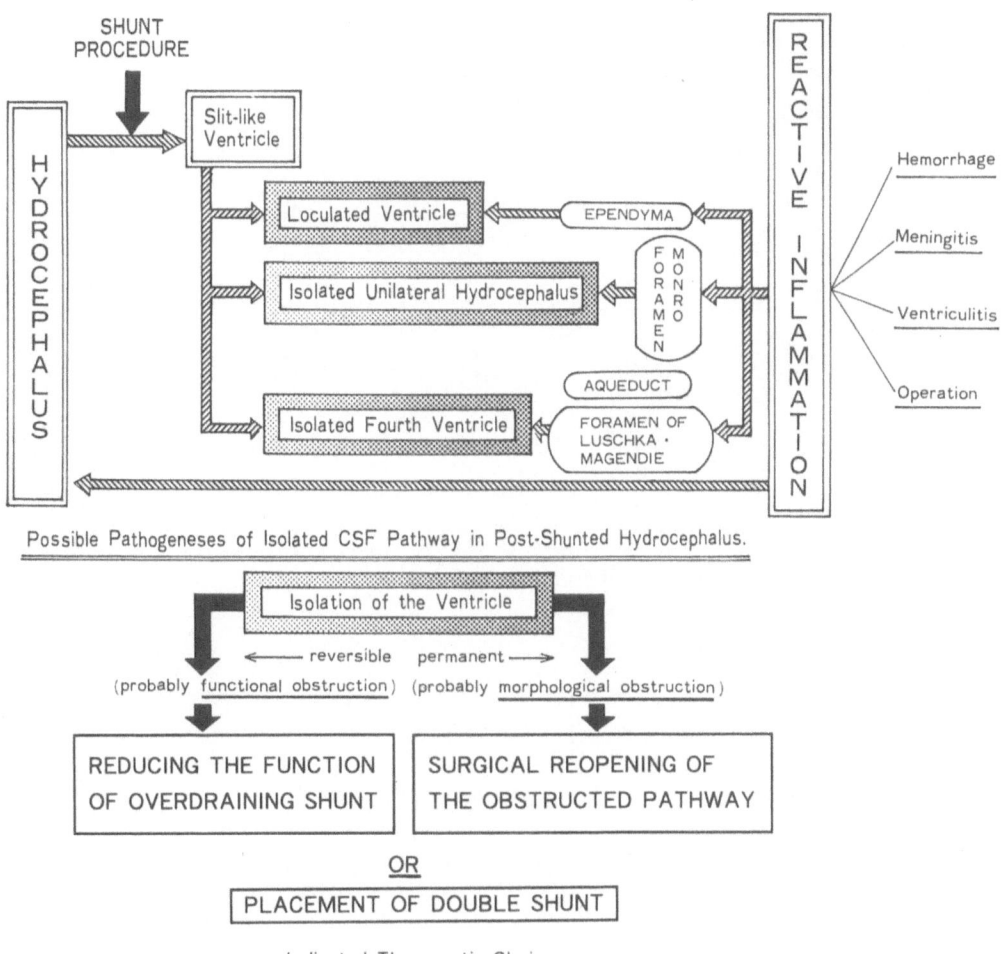

Figure 2. Possible pathophysiology of post-shunt isolated ventricles and therapeutic choice (Oi and Matsumoto).

VI) Follow-up and Long-term Result

Statistical Analysis of Influencial Factors on Prognosis of Hydrocephalic Patients

Satoshi Matsumoto, Takashi Tsubokawa, Yutaka Maki, Kiyoshi Satoh, Shouzou Ishii, Katsutoshi Kitamura, Norihiko Tamaki, and Mitsuru Kimura

The Research Committee of "Hydrocephalus," The Ministry of Health and Welfare of Japan

Authors performed clinical study to analyze statistically the therapeutic problems and factors on the hydrocephalic patients, especially of the case resisting against treatment. Statistical studies consist of analysis on 145 cases of hydrocephalus (Evan's ratio<30%) which admitted to neurosurgical institutes in Japan (43 institutes) from January 1984 to December 1986. All patient was monitored its intracranial pressure and the pressure was less than 180 mmH$_2$O. Patients were devided into 3 groups by their post operative conditions (exellent, good, unchanged or worse). Statistical studies were used by X^2 test.

87 (60%) cases are male and 58(40%) cases are female. The age is ranged from 28 to 81 (mean=61.04, S.D.=11.97).

(Causes of hydrocephalus): (*Table 1*)

(Operations): Operated cases 127 (V-P shunt 117, L-P shunt 10). Non-operated cases 18.

(Result of statistical analysis): Some factors are statistically significant. Post operative recovery rate of dementia between non-traumatic (post subarachnoid hemorrhage) hydrocephalus and idiopathic hydrocephalus is statistically significant as *Table 2*. Idiopathic hydrocephalus was more resistent against treatment than the other. Hydrocephalus with brain atrophy is the most resistent factor against treatment (*Table 3*). Continuous intracranial pressure monitoring was useful. High steady state pressure is the factor of good response to treatment (*Figure*). Intracranial pressure monitoring by single tap method is not so useful.

(Annual Report of the Research Committee of "Hydrocephalus," The Ministry of Health and Welfare of Japan, 1986: 199–206, 1987)

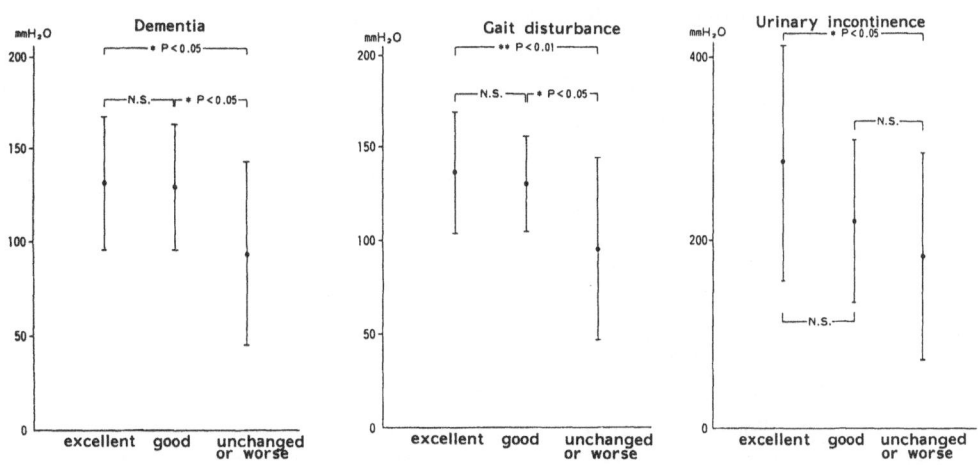

Figure. Relationship between base line I.C.P. and post operative conditions.

Key words: Hydrocephalus, Normal pressure hydrocephalus, Statistical analysis

Table 1.

Cases	Cases	%
non-traumatic intra-cerebral or intra-ventricular hemorrhage	11	7.59
traumatic intra-cerebral or intra-ventricular hemorrhage	1	0.69
non-traumatic subarachnoid hemorrhage	61	42.07
traumatic subarachnoid hemorrhage	3	2.07
non-traumatic subdural hemorrhage	1	0.69
traumatic subdural hemorrhage	0	0.00
meningitis	4	2.76
idiopathic	50	34.48
others	10	6.90
unknown	4	2.74
Total	145	100.00

Table 2.

(Dementia)

	Idiopathic	Non-traumatic SAH	Total
excellent	3	18	21
good	10	23	33
unchanged or worse	23	10	33
Total	36	51	87

(**P<0.01)

(Gait disturbance)

	Idiopathic	Non-traumatic SAH	Total
excellent	8	19	27
good	11	16	27
unchanged or worse	16	18	34
Total	35	53	88

(N.S)

(Urinary incontinence)

	Idiopathic	Non-traumatic SAH	Total
excellent	6	22	28
good	4	12	16
unchanged or worse	24	16	40
Total	34	50	84

(**P<0.01)

Table 3.

(Dementia)

	Atrophy (−)	Atrophy (mild)	Atrophy (severe)	Total
excellent	19	8	2	29
good	21	22	3	46
unchanged or worse	9	24	11	44
Total	49	54	16	119

(**P<0.01)

(Gait disturbance)

	Atrophy (−)	Atrophy (mild)	Atrophy (severe)	Total
excellent	24	10	2	36
good	15	16	3	34
unchanged or worse	11	28	11	50
Total	50	54	16	120

(**P<0.01)

(Urinary incontinence)

	Atrophy (−)	Atrophy (mild)	Atrophy (severe)	Total
excellent	20	12	2	34
good	13	10	2	25
unchanged or worse	14	30	12	56
Total	47	52	16	115

(*P<0.05)

Prognostic Signs in Fetal Hydrocephalus

Willy Serlo,[1] Pertti Kirkinen,[2] Pentti Jouppila,[2] and Riitta Herva[3]

[1]Department of Pediatrics, [2]Department of Obstetrics and Gynecology, and [3]Department of Pathology, University of Oulu, Oulu, Finland

An antenatal diagnosis of fetal hydrocephalus was made in 38 cases. Using certain criteria for the assessment of fetal prognosis, 23 cases were considered to be deverely affected. Postnatal evaluation of these 23 cases established the extensive severity of fetal abnormality in all cases. The prognosis was estimated to be more favorable in 10 cases, of which 8 were delivered by elective cesarean section and 2 by spontaneous vaginal delivery. In 9 cases a ventriculoarterial shunting procedure was performed early in the neonatal period, while 1 case was treated conservatively. Follow-up of these 10 cases (at 7 months to 5 years of age) revealed normal or subnormal development in 6 cases and severe retardation in 4. Fetal hydrocephalus proved to have several etiological causes and was associated with other anomalies in 84% of cases. Severe forms of fetal hydrocephalus can, by means of modern ultrasound techniques, be detected before the 20th gestational week. Some cases of fetal hydrocephalus progress slowly during the fetal period. These can be followed until term by repeated ultrasound examinations and good or moderate prognosis can be expected with the use of early postnatal therapy. Only a minority of hydrocephalic fetuses seem to be potential objects for antenatal shunting.   (Child's Nerv Syst 2: 93–97, 1986)

Key words: Congenital hydrocephalus, Antenatal diagnosis, Ultrasound

Table. Prognostically poor signs at ultrasound evaluation of the hydrocephalic fetus

Findings associated with fetal hydrocephaly
Multiple extracranial anomalies
Severe intracranial anomaly (*i.e.* holoporencephaly, missing midline structure, large tumor, or agenesis of the cerebellum)
Severe fetal growth retardation
No recognizable cortex, even at the thalamic level
Retarded (microcephalic) cranial growth (biparietal diameter or circumference)

Long Term Follow Up Study of Spina Bifida Cystica

Masahiro IZAWA

Department of Neurosurgery, Neurological Institute, Tokyo Women's Medical College, Tokyo, Japan

In the past 15 years, 32 cases of the spina bifida cystica were experienced. We have made a long-term follow-up study of these cases as correlated with the hydrocephalus.
Not a few cases of the spina bifida cystica are seen accompanying a variety of complications. The hydrocephalus, in particular, has a strong possibility of seriously affecting the prognosis of mentality. Out of 32 cases there were 22 cases where the complication with hydrocephalus was observed. Prognosis of mentality heavily depends on the therapeutic performance on this

complication. In some cases the paraparensis or disturbance of the bladder and rectum remain as a sequella after operation.

In the MRI study, which was made as part of our follow-up diagnosis for post operative consideration should be given to these cases in the early operation, as there is a strong possibility that tethered cord may result in the functional disturbance of the patients. MRI is applicable to child outpatients and is considered useful.

(Shoni no Noshinkei 11: 447–451, 1986)

Key words: Spina bifida cystica, Hydrocephalus, MRI

Table.   Preceding reconstructing operation

(I)

A)

reconstructing operation	case	mental state		
less 24 hs.	5	A(3) B(2)		
24 hs. to 48 hs.	3	A(2)	D(1)	
48 hs. to 1 w.	5	A(3) B(1)		E(1)
1 w. to 1 m.	6	A(6)		
more 1 m.	6	A(4) C(2)		

B)

operation (−)	6		D(2) E(4)

C)

unknown	1	B(1)

total	32	A(18) B(4) C(2) D(3) E(5)

(II)

A)

liquorrhea group	case	mental state		
a) hydrocephalus (−)	2	A(2)		
b) hydrocephalus (+)	14	A(7) B(2)		D(2) E(3)
·shunt after reconstruction				
before 2 wks. (7)		A(6)		D(1)
2 wks. to 1 m. (2)		A(1) B(1)		
1 m. to 3 ms. (1)		B(1)		
·no reconstruction				
shunt only (2)				D(1) E(1)
·no reconstruction				
no shunt (2)				E(2)

B)

no liquorrhea group	12		
a) hydrocephalus (−) (8)		A(8)	
b) hydrocephalus (+) (4)		A(3) C(1)	

C)

unknown	4

(A: normal, B: debility, C: imbecility, D: idiocy).

Prognostic Significance of Signs and Symptoms in Hydrocephalus: Analysis of survival

Jette JANSEN and Merete JØRGENSEN

Department of Neurosurgery and Paediatrics, Uneversity Hospital, Copenhagen and Statistical Research Unit, Danish Medical and Social Science Research Councils, Copenhagen, Denmark

Using Cox's regression model, an analysis was made to identify signs and symptoms of prognostic significance in hydrocephalic infants and young children. The material consists of 231 patients born between 1946 and 1955 with hydrocephalus diagnosed or suspected before the age of five years (87% before 2 years). The material was collected retrospectively. Age at follow-up was 21 to 35 years.

The model used in the statistical analysis allows for different times of entry and makes it possible to analyse the effects of several covariates. The influence of a given covariate is expressed by a factor of excess mortality. The necessary assumption for doing this is that the death intensities for all patients are proportional.

The covariates included were sex, complications during pregnancy and birth, birth weight and year of first admission (constant covariates) and signs of hydrocephalus, treatment, seizures and duration (time-dependent covariates). The inclusion of time-dependent covariates is an extension of the model, whereby the dynamics of the condition can be analysed.

The only constant covariate of prognostic importance was asphyxia with a factor of excess mortality of 1.70. Important time-dependent covariates were: a head circumference increasingly above the 97th percentile and/or a radiological diagnosis of hydrocephalus, general seizures and a short lapse of time since diagnosis, the factors of excess mortality ranging from 2.5 to 6.3.

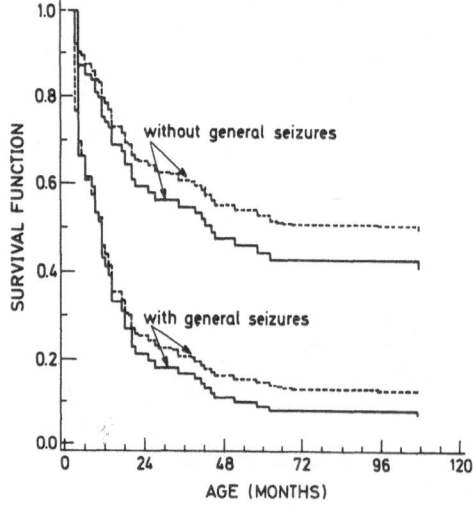

Figure. Patients admitted at age one month with and without general seizures.
Without downward-displaced eyes (---) and with downward-displaced eyes (—).

An excess mortality of patients with the sign of downward-displaced eyes (occurring before the sunset sign) could not be expressed by a factor, because the excess mortality was age-dependent (death intensities not proportional).

Application of the model to individual patients requires access to an alectronic data system. By entering the data of the individual patient, a survival curve can be obtained that takes into consideration the characteristics of that patient.   (Acta Neurol Scand 73: 55–65, 1986)

Key words: Cox regression model, Excess mortality, Prognosis

Ventriculoperitoneal Shunts in Low Birth Weight Infants with Intracranial Hemorrhage:
Neurodevelopmental outcome

Bruce R. Boynton, Carole A. Boynton, T. Allen Merritt, Yvonne E. Vaucher, Hector E. James, and Raul F. Bejar

Division of Neonatal/Perinatal Medicine and Division of Neurosurgery, Department of Pediatrics, University of California, San Diego, School of Medicine, San Diego, California, USA

Fifty preterm infants (mean birth weight, 1266±303 g; mean gestational age, 30±2 weeks) who required a ventriculoperitoneal (VP) shunt for posthemorrhagic hydrocephalus (92% with Grade III or IV hemorrhage) were followed for neurodevelopmental problems. VP shunts were placed at a median age of 29 days (range, 18 to 87 days) after serial lumbar punctures failed to control progressive and symptomatic ventriculomegaly. A total of 34 infants (68%) required one shunt revision or more (median, 4 revisions) for infection or obstruction. Shunt infection occurred in 25 infants (50%) after initial placement or revision for a gross operative infection rate of 18.8%. Seven infants died, 2 from shunt infections. The infants were evaluated with audiological, ophthalmological, and neurodevelopmental examinations. Of the survivors, 11 (28%) have severe visual loss, 10 (24%) have hearing loss, and 4 (11%) have impairment of both senses. Of the infants, 21 (49%) have significant paralysis or muscle weakness, 19 (38%) have seizure disorders, and 7 (16%) are microcephalic. Developmental and motor scores were obtained using the Bayley or Knobloch-Gesell scales at 2, 6, 12, 18 and 24 months of age. Both developmental and motor scores were normal in 7 of the surviving infants (18%). Sixteen infants (41%) have one abnormal score and in 16 infants (41%) both developmental and motor scores were abnormal, indicating profound developmental delay. Twenty-six of the survivors (60%) have multiple handicaps. There was no association between developmental or motor scores and the number of shunt infections or revisions. Grade IV hemorrhage or the occurrence of repeated seizures was a predictor of poor neurodevelopmental outcome. We conclude that early VP shunt placement is feasible and effective in controlling symptomatic posthemorrhagic hydrocephalus in low birth weight infants. However, the data indicate that early shunt placement is still associated with a high incidence of neurodevelopmental abnormalities.

(Neurosurgery 18: 141–145, 1986)

Key words: Hydrocephalus, Intraventricular hemorrhage, Newborn, Ventriculoperitoneal shunt

Table. Distribution of developmental scores

Category	Score	Developmental Score	Motor Score
Severely delayed	<52	18 (46%)	21 (54%)
Moderately delayed	52–83	9 (23%)	10 (26%)
Normal	>83	12 (31%)	8 (21%)

Developmental Outcome of Infants with Severe Intracranial-intraventricular Hemorrhage and Hydrocephalus with and without Ventriculoperitoneal Shunt

P. Sasidharan, E. Marquez, E. Dizon, and C. V. Sridhar

Department of Neonatology, Porter Memorial Hospital, Indiana University, Valparaiso, IN, USA

Intraventricular hemorrhage continues to be a major contributor to significant morbidity in surviving very low birth weight infants. It is not clear, whether ventriculomegaly that frequently follows severe IVH (grades III and IV) or the severity and the extent of the hemorrhage itself is responsible for the subsequent developmental sequelae.

We studied the developmental outcome of 36 infants (mean birth weight 1240±498 gms and gestational age 29.1 weeks, range 24–40 weeks) who developed grade III or IV intraventricular hemorrhage during their neonatal period, comparing the outcome of infants with and without ventriculo-peritoneal shunts. All these infants had ventriculomegaly and were treated with serial lumbar punctures for upto two weeks. 15 infants (41.6%) required VP shunts because of progressive enlargement of the ventricles after the daily lumbar punctures were discontinued. Using Denver developmental and Bayley scales, the developmental quotient was determined. DQ is the value of the functioning age divided by the chronological age (corrected for prematurity)/100. DQ of >85 was considered normal; DQ of <75 was considered abnormal and DQs between 75 to 85 as suspect group. Fifty percent of the total group of infants had normal developmental quotient (DQ>85). The mean developmental quotient of the infants who did not require VPS was 88.71 and of the group who required VPS was 67.93 (P<.02). Among the nonshunted (NVPS) group 61.9% (13/21) had developmental quotients greater than 85 (normal), while among the shunted (VPS) group only 33.3% (5/15) had DQ greater than 85 by a mean chronological age of 16.25+7.5 months (corrected age of 14 months). Similarly, among the VPS group 46.6% and among the non-VPS group 19.05% had abnormal DQ (<75). All infants with VPS survived and in two cases shunt revisions were carried out because of shunt blockage. Our results indicate that infants, who develop posthemorrhagic hydrocephalus requiring VP shunts had a poorer developmental outcome, compared to those infants who did not require shunts. Those infants whose ventricular size became normal after VP shunts had a normal outcome in our series. This might be due to the fact that these infants did not suffer periventricular infarction which is a major factor in determining the neurodevelopmental outcome.

(Child's Nerv Syst 2: 149–152, 1986)

Key words: Intraventricular hemorrhage, Developmental quotient, Ventriculoperitoneal shunt, Ventriculomegaly, Hydrocephalus

Table. Results of the follow-up data and characteristics of the two groups of infants with and without VP shunt

	VP Shunt (N=15 mean±SD)	Non-VP Shunt (N=21 mean±SD)	P
Developmental quotient	67.93± 26.5	88.71± 22.07	<0.02
Chronological age	15.53± 8.47	16.76± 7.4	NS
Corrected age	13.3 ± 9.1	14.51± 8.35	NS
Birth/weight (grams)	1,243.3 ±631.9	1,237.6 ±395	NS
Age (weeks)	29 ± 4.1	29.28± 2.95	NS
PH	7.20	7.20	NS
PCO$_2$	52.2	55.6	NS
Apgar (1 min)	4	4.4	NS
Apgar (5 min)	5.7	6	NS

Motor Disturbances in Normal-pressure Hydrocephalus:
Special reference to stance and gait

Per Soelberg Sørensen, Erik C. Jansen, and Flemming Gjerris

University Clinics of Neurology and Neurosurgery, Rigshospitalet, Copenhagen, and Biomechanical Laboratorium, Copenhagen County Hospital, Gentofte, Denmark

Motor disturbances were studied in 16 patients with normal-pressure hydrocephalus (NPH) before and 3 to 6 months after shunt operation. All patients had a history of progressive dementia, gait disturbances, and urinary incontinence; hydrocephalus, defined as Evans' ratio above 0.30 in CT; mean intraventricular pressure below 12 mm Hg during 24–48 pressure monitoring; and decreased conductance to CSF outflow measured by lumbo-ventricular perfusion.

Motor performance in the upper extremities was assessed by handwriting test, peg-board test, and hand-tremor measurement using an accelerometer. Postural instability was measured on a computer-assisted force-plate, and computerized analysis of gait was made using an instrumented treadmill. All results were compared with measurements in age-matched controls.

Table. Effect of shunt operation on stance and gait in 12 patients with NPH*

	Before Shunt Operation	After Shunt Operation
Stance		
Sway with open eyes, cm·10^{-2}	114 (47)	80 (32)+
Sway with closed eyes, cm·10^{-2}	138 (3)	100 (44)+
Gait		
Stance phase, % of stride	69 (3)	67 (2)+
Double support time, % of stride	37 (3)	34 (3)+
Stride length, cm	50 (22)	61 (18)+
Speed of gait, km/hr	1.6 (0.7)	1.9 (0.6)+
Ataxia‡		
Left vertical	11.0 (4.1)	6.8 (1.9)+
Left transversal	1.3 (0.8)	0.9 (0.2)+
Left sagittal	2.6 (1.0)	1.9 (0.4)+
Total	30.1 (13.3)	18.4 (4.0)+

* NPH indicates normal-pressure hydrocephalus. Values in parentheses are SDs.
+ $p<.5$ compared with values before shunt operation.
‡ Force as percentage of body weight.

was significantly increased in NPH patients (140 ± 11 cm$\cdot10^{-2}$) compared with controls (93 ± 6 cm$\cdot10^{-2}$) ($p<0.01$). The gait of the NPH patients was characterized by a very low speed and short stride length compared with controls. The ataxia or unsteadiness of gait was increased, especially in the vertical direction, and calculation of the external work per meter of gait showed that walking was much more energy consuming in patients with NPH than in controls.

After shunt operation the speed of handwriting, peg-board time and tremor intensity improved but were still significantly inferior to the controls. The effect of shunt operation on stance and gait is shown in the table. After shunting the postural instability and the total gait ataxia were within the 95% confidence interval for controls.

In conclusion, the study shows that many of the severe motor disturbances in NPH can be relieved by shunt operation. (Arch Neurol 43: 34–38, 1986)

Key words: Ataxia, Postural instability, Computerized gait analysis, Shunt-operation

Prognosis of Dementia in Normal-pressure Hydrocephalus after a Shunt Operation

A. M. Thomsen, S. E. Børgesen, P. Bruhn, and F. Gjerris

Department of Neurosurgery and Section of Neuropsychology, Rigshospitalet, Copenhagen, Denmark

Dementia in NPH is a state which is generally accepted as being reversible after shunting. The reversibility is seldom demonstrated by adequate objective methods. In the present investigation 40 patients with a diagnosis of NPH were neuropsychologically examined before and 12 months after a ventriculo-atrial shunt operation. Comparison of the pre- and postoperative test results showed that cognitive functions improved in 16 patients, were unchanged in 19, and deteriorated in 5.

Analysis of the test results showed that improvement took place especially in vigilance, measured by a reaction time test. Visuospatial functions also improved, but not secondary to the improved vigilance.

Moreover, we found that the outcome of the shunt operation depended on selection criteria. Patients with NPH of known cause had a far better treatment outcome than did those with idiopathic NPH. It is tempting to conclude that idiopathic NPH is beyond the reach of surgical correction.

However, our improvement criteria were conservative. A more liberal improvement criterion might have included those patients in whom the shunt procedure stopped further deterioration, *i.e.* patients with an unchanged postoperative neuropsychological level. This was the case in 14 of our patients with NPH of unknown etiology, and it cannot be ruled out that progressive deterioration was arrested by surgical intervention in these patients. Apart from known cause, short history, low cerebrospinal fluid outflow, small sulci and/or periventricular hypodensity were also found to be favourable selection criteria. With three or more of these preoperative signs being present, improvement in cognitive functions was seen in 80% of the patients after shunt operation.   (Ann Neurol 20: 304–310, 1986)

Key words: Normal-pressure hydrocephalus (NPH), Prognosis, Shunt operation, Dementia, Neuropsychological testing

Table. Preoperative clinical and investigational variables in relation to postoperative improvement in the neuropsychological examination

Preoperative Variable	N	Improved	P^a
Age			
<60	24	10	NS
≥60	16	6	
Cause			
Known	21	14	<0.01
Unknown	19	2	
Length of history (mo)			
3–6	14	9	
6–12	7	4	<0.05
12–24	4	0	
>24	15	3	
Evans ratio			
≥0.40	11	6	NS
<0.40	29	10	
Periventricular edema			
Present	11	9	=0.01
Absent	29	7	
Sulci on CT			
Small (<2.0mm)	12	11	
Normal	14	3	<0.01
Dilated (>5.0mm)	14	2	
C_{out} (ml/min/mm Hg)			
0–0.05	18	11	
0.051–0.08	15	4	<0.02
0.081–0.12	7	1	

[a] Fischer's Exact Test.
CT=computed tomography;   NS=not   significant;
C_{out}=outflow of cerebrospinal fluid.

Gait Analysis in Patients with Normal Pressure Hydrocephalus: Its dynamic characteristics and tracks to better rehabilitation methodology

Itaru KIMURA, Shun-ichi SASO, Ayumu OHNUMA, and Taisuke OHTSUKI

Neurological Research Center, Miyagi National Hospital, Miyagi, Japan

The gait disturbance in patients with normal pressure hydrocephalus (NPH) has not analysed in detail, because of its complexity. The purpose of the study was to delineate the mechanism of the gait disturbance in NPH patients, using a modern gait analysis system and to find tracks of effective physical therapy for better gait ability.

Subjects consisted 5 NPH patients diagnosed clinically and confirmed by metrazemide CT scan and 50 healthy volunteers, ages ranged from 18 to 79. With a force-plate system following 6 parameters were analysed. (1) Fz=mean vertical force calculated as a body weight taken as 100%, (2) Fz (R/L)=right and left vertical force ratio calculated as a left Fz taken as 100%, (3) Fx%=lateral forces determined as a Fz taken as 100%, (4) Fy%=antero-posterior forces calculated as a Fz taken as 100%, (5) D.S.P.=double stance phase, and (6) S.P.=single stance phase were obtained. To evaluate the walking posture, graphic display of foot to ground pressure distribution and sequences of joint angle of each

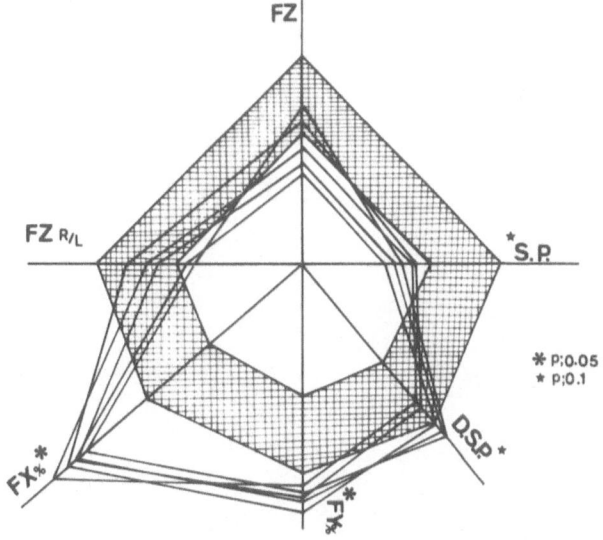

Figure. Gait dynamic characteristics in patients with normal pressure hydrocephalus and 50 normal subjects (*shaded area*) displayed in 6 parameters obtained with forceplate system. Fz=vertical forces, Fx%=lateral force ratio, Fy%=antero-posterior force ratio, DSP=double stance phase and SP=single stance phase.

lower extremity during gait were recorded simultaneously.

Gait characteristics in patients with NPH were summarized in *Figure*. (1) Fx% was significantly increased ($p<0.01$), which indicated that patients swang irregularly to both sides, (2) Fy% was significantly increased ($p<0.005$), which suggested decomposition between initial kick and terminal brake seen in normal gait pattern, (3) double stance phase was prolonged with irregularly shortened single stance phase, which might suggest "magnetic apraxia of gait" described clinically.

These gait characteristics lead us clues to effective physical therapy. (1) To enhance the somatosensory input from the feet and joints, weighted shoes was sometimes effective to stabilize the body balance. (2) balance and rhythm training, and (3) enhancement of rude power in the lower extremities might be essential.

(Annual Report of the Research Committee "Progressive Hydrocephalus," The Ministry of Health and Welfare of Japan, 1986: 183–188, 1987)

Key words: Progressive hydrocephalus, Gait analysis, Rehabilitation

VII) Classification of Hydrocephalus

Congenital
  Cranium bifidum and spina bifida
  Holoprosencephaly
  Foramen atresia
  Congenital cyst
  Others
Acquired
  Brain tumor
  Hemorrhagic or other vascular diseases
  Infection
Normal Pressure Hydrocephalus

Follow-up Study of Selective Early Operation for Myelomeningocele

Hiroshi NISHIMOTO, Takashi TSUBOKAWA, and Saburo NAKAMURA

Department of Neurological Surgery, Nihon University School of Medicine, Tokyo, Japan

During 1975–81, 40 infants with myelomeningocele were treated in our clinic. 36 of 40 cases, considered to have favorable prognosis by Stein's selection protocol, were selected for back closure and vigorous subsequent treatment. All of these cases which survived were followed up for two years or more after operation and we investigated the prognosis in 1983. In this paper, long-term follow-up results of survivors after operation were assessed.

Four cases with open myelomeningocele died of serious prulent meningitis within 1 month after admission. 30 of 36 operated cases with open or closed myelomeningocele survived during the follow-up period. Among these survivors, 21 cases with open myelomeningocele were less severely handicapped. 80% of these 21 cases were ambulatory with or whithout aids and 70% of these cases had IQs of 80 or above. 40% of these cases had incontinence with dilatation of the upper urinary tracts revealed by pyelogram. Among these 21 infants with open myelomeningocele, 15 infants had early surgery within the first 48 hours of life and 6 had delayed surgery between 3 and 7 days of age. Survival rates were similar between these two groups and no significant association existed between the time of surgery and development of ventriculitis, or prognosis.

Seven infants with open myelomeningocele had one of Lorber's adverse criteria on admission. These seven cases had more severe handicaps in locomotion, urinary tracts and intelligence, in contrast with the cases who didn't have any of Lorber's criteria which had less severe handicaps. However 43% of 7 cases with Lorber's criteria had IQs of 80 or above at the end of the follow-up period.

In 5 cases with open myelomeningocele, lacunar skull deformities were revealed on craniogram before back closures. All 5 of the cases with lacunar skull deformity had hydrocephalus. But there was no striking association between the lacunar skull deformity and the grade of hydrocephalus, or follow-up results of intelligence. None of the 5 infants had severe mental or developmental retardation during the follow-up period.

It might be concluded that early back closure within the first 48 hours of life and lacunar skull deformity revealed on craniogram are less important for the prognosis than reported previously in infants with open myelomeningocele.   (*Shoni no Noshinkei* 11: 307–313, 1986)

Key words: Myelomeningocele, Spina bifida, Hydrocephalus, Selective operation

Table. Follow-up results in survived operative 21 cases with open myelomeningocele

Follow-up results	Time of operation (back closure)	
	within 48 hours after birth 15 cases	more than 3rd day of life 6 cases
Level of lesion		
L_3-	2 (13%)	1 (17%)
$-L_4$	6 (40)	1 (17)
$-S_1$	7 (47)	2 (33)
$-S_3$	0 (—)	2 (33)
Hydrocephalus		
Present	13 (87)	5 (83)
Absent	2 (13)	1 (17)
Complications		
Infection		
Present	2 (13)	2 (33)
Absent	13 (87)	4 (67)
Revision No. of shunt		
0	3	0
1–2	6	3
3–	4	2
Outcome*		
Locomotion		
Grade 0	3 (20)	1 (17)
1	1 (7)	1 (17)
2	3 (20)	1 (17)
3	8 (53)	3 (50)
Sphincter involvement		
Grade 0	6 (40)	1 (17)
1	4 (27)	0 (—)
2	3 (20)	1 (17)
3	2 (13)	4 (67)
Intelligence		
Grade 0	1 (7)	0 (—)
1	3 (20)	2 (33)
2	11 (73)	4 (67)

*1. Assessments of locomotion

Grade 0 complete paralysis, wheel chair
    1 walking with aids
    2 walking without aids
    3 walking normally

2. Assessments of sphincter involvement

Grade 0 incontinence, abnormal renal function
    1 crede, clean intermittent catheterization dilatation in the upper urinary tracts
    2 crede, clean intermittent catheterization normal upper urinary tracts
    3 normal

3. Assessments of intelligence

Grade 0 IQ or DQ<60
    1   60–80
    2   >80

Lobar Holoprosencephaly with Hydrocephalus:
Antenatal demonstration and differential diagnosis

Janet C. Hoffman-Tretin,[1] Dikran S.Horoupian,[2] Mordecai Koenigsberg,[1] Michael J. Schnur,[1] Josephine R. Llena[2]

Departments of [1]Radiology and [2]Pathology, Albert Einstein College of Medicine, Bronx Municipal Hospital Center, Bronx, New York, USA

Two proven cases of lobar holoprosencephaly with hydrocephalus and·on likely but unproven case were studied in utero by sonography. Characteristic sonographic features were defind which corresponded to known anatomic and CT features of this entity. These include incomplete anterior falx, absence of the septum pellucidum and corpus callosum, apparent marked hydrocephalus with little parietoccipital mantle (representing in part a "dorsal" cyst), abnormal thalami, and superior and anterior blunting of the frontal horns. Differential diagnostic considerations for lobar holoprosencephaly with hydrocephalus include simple obstructive hydrocephalus (aqueductal stenosis, etc.) and various cystic intracranial malformations. Lobar holoprosencephaly is the least severe of a spectrum of cerebral malformations resulting from·incomplete division of the embryonic prosencephalon into two hemispheres.

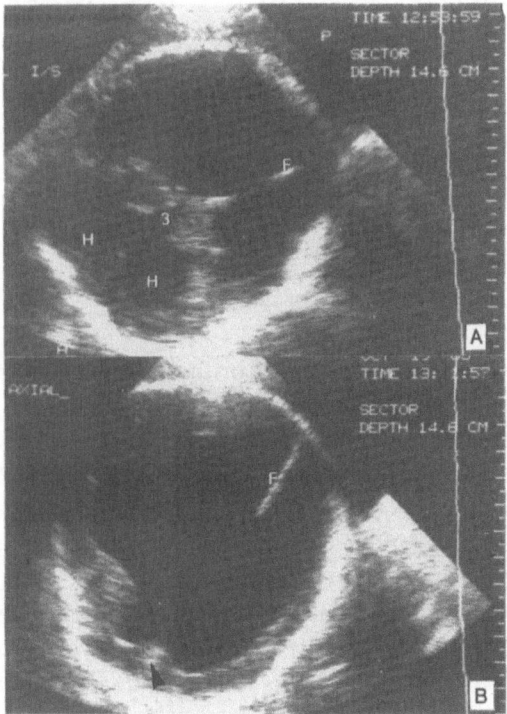

Figure. Case 2. Lobar holoprosencephaly with hydrocephalus in a 32 week gestation. **A** (*top*), axial view of the fetal head shows posterior falx (F), confluent dysplastic frontal horns (H), and third ventricle (3). **B** (*bottom*), on a higher axial section, the confluent ventricular structures are interrupted by a posterior segment of falx (F), which is eccentric in position. Frontal lobation is suggested by apparent anterior interhemispheric fissure (*arrow*) and shallow blunted frontal horns.

It may be distinguished from the more severe forms of holoprosencephal alobar and semilobar, by the presence of a common lateral ventricle in the first and fusion of the anterior horns in the second. In hydranencephaly, cerebral mantle is absent or demonstrable only in the occipital regions. Agenesis of the corpus callosum with associated interhemispheric cyst and septooptic dysplasia may be indistinguishable from lobar holoprosencephaly by imaging alone. The sonographic features of agenesis of the corpus callosum include widely separated slit-like frontal horns as well as widely separated ventricular bodies with a characteristic medial concavity. Obstructive hydrocephalus, which may carry the best prognosis, is characterized by clearly defined frontal horns and preservation of frontal mantle.

Precise antenatal diagnoses of intracranial anomalies is important because of differences in prognosis and resulting implications for obstetric management as well as genetic counseling. The prognosis for alobar and semilobar holoprosencephaly as well as hydranencephaly is dismal. Lobar holoprosencephaly, like agenesis of the corpus callosum with associated cerebral anomaly, has a variable prognosis but frequently results in mental retardation.

(J Ultrasound Med 5: 691–697, 1986)

Key words: Ultrasonography, Obstetric; Fetus(es), Congenital anomalies; Holoprosencephaly, Lobar

A Case of Holoprosencephaly with Atypical CT Findings and No Facial Anomaly

Eiichiro Honda, Takashi Hayashi, Kazuto Shojima, Takao Shojima, and Sinken Kuramoto

Department of Neurosurgery, St. Mary's Hospital, Kurume, Japan

Holoprosencephaly is generally thought to be an anomaly due to a growth disturbance in the process of differentiation of the prosencephalon in the 5th week of the embryonic stage. The diagnosis of this disease only by CT scan is extremely difficult except in typical cases. There are cases of holoprosencephaly which are misdiagnosed as extensive subdural effusion on CT scan, being without facial anomaly such as hare lip, cleft palate and hypotelorism.

We report a case of a 3 month old female infant, presenting with an increased tension of the fontanelle, cramp and irritability. No abnormality was noted during the periods of her mother's pregnancy and delivery. Although the CT findings in this case apparently revealed seemingly the pattern of severe subdural effusion, the cerebral ventricle was proved to be single. Cerebral angiography showed the anterior cerebral artery running along the frontal base. The Sylvian triangle was not formed in the arterial phase. In the venous phase, the superior sagittal sinus was formed incompletely. Deep cerebral veins (straight sinus internal cerebral and the Galen veins) were not visualized although a variety of abnormal vein net works were observed. Holoprosencephaly was diagnosed this time. In this case, the histological findings at the operation confirmed that the subdural effusion-like space on CT was actually the dorsal sac.

From this case, two important points are that (1) as Demyer mentioned, this case was compatible with the morphology of holoprosecephaly in that cerebral parenchyma was retroflexed in a posterior direction. The phenomenon of retroflexion may be explained by the finding that the formation of the bridging vein, which normally drain blood to the superior sagittal sinus and protect the cerebral parenchyma from shifting, are incomplete in holoprosencephaly because the superior sagittal sinus is hypoplastic or in defective in this anomaly, (2) The patient did not show any facial malformation. The CT findings were also atypical appearence. The definite diagnosis was, therefore, made possible only by cerebral angiography.   (*Shoni no Noshinkei* 11: 117–122, 1986)

Key words: Holoprosencephaly, Cerebral angiography, Subdural effusion, Dorsal sac, Retroflexion

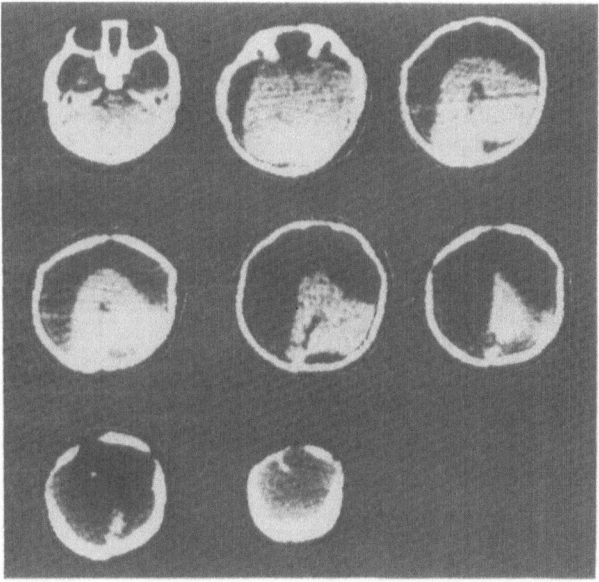

Figure.   Subdural effusion was suspected on CT scan. The supraventricular system was monoventricle. Dorsal Sac (low density area) was observed at the posterior of the skull.

An Autopsy Case of Holoprosencephaly with Endocrine Abnormalities

Yumi Horigome,[1] Kenzo Hamano,[1] Hiroshi Kanma,[2] Kenji Shin,[1] Hitoshi Takita,[1] and Takesaburo Ogata[2]

Departments of [1]Pediatrics, and [2]Pathology, University of Tsukuba, Ibaraki, Japan

We experienced a case of holoprosencephaly associated with endocrine abnormalities. A male neonate, one of twins, was born at 36 weeks of gestation. The other twin had no abnormalities. At birth, our case weighed 2,780g, had dyspnea and was immediately intubated. He had a single nostril, ocular hypotelorism and small ophthalmus. CT scan showed a single ventricle and a large dorsal sack, which suggested the diagnosis of holoprosencephaly. He died 26 hours after birth because of respiratory failure. Autopsy was performed and semilobar type of holoprosencephaly was confirmed. The pituitary gland was completely absent. The adrenal cortex and thyroid gland exhibited severe atrophy (20% and 36% of normal size, respectively). There was no colloid formation of the thyroid gland. Bilateral testes were not descended but their sizes and histological findings were normal. The serum pituitary hormones were examined. Their values were as follows: GH 1.7ng/m*l* (normal: 10–40), TSH less than 1.0uU/m*l* (normal: 3–18), FSH 10.6 mIU/m*l* (normal: 0–21.5) and LH 11.3 mIU/m*l* (normal: 3.1–5.2). GH and TSH levels were very low, but FSH and LH showed normal values.

In the 1950's Yakovlev and Edmonds reported that holoprosencephaly frequently accompa-

Table. Endocrine abnormalities in holoprosencephaly of the cases in literatures and our case

	Haworth[1]		Hintz[2]		Begleiter[3]	Our case
	Case 1	Case 3	Case 1	Case 2	Case 2	
pituitary gland	absent	absent	absent	unknown (alive)	absent	absent
adrenal gland	atrophied (0.5g)	atrophied (2.1g)	atrophied (0.5g)		atrophied (1g)	atrophied (1.4g)
thyroid gland	hypoplasia (0.46g)	normal	N.D.		N.D.	hypoplasia (0.65)
testis/ovary	N.D.	normal	N.D.		N.D.	normal
GH				normal		low
TSH	N.E.	N.E.	N.E.	normal	N.E.	low
ACTH				low		N.E.
FSH				N.E.		normal
LH				N.E.		normal
ADH				low		N.E.

[1] J Pediatr 1961; 59: 726–33. [2] J Pediatr 1968; 72: 81–7. [3] Am J Med Genet 1980; 7: 315–8. (N.E.: not examined, N.D.: not described).

nies the agenesis of pituitary gland. However, there was only slight knowledge of the values of serum pituitary hormones and other endocrinological abnormalities. In the present case, the adrenal cortex and thyroid gland were atrophied but the testicular gland was normal. This was consistent with the fact that serum GH and TSH were lowered but LH and FSH were normally secreted. From these findings we concluded that this case had an ectopic pituitary gland. We also considered that prosencephaly and pituitary gland dysgenesis simultaneous had occurred simultaneously at 3 to 5 weeks of gestation, resulting in hypoplasia of thyroid and adrenal glands.

(No to Hattatsu 18: 228–233, 1986)

Key words: Holoprosencephaly, Endocrine abnormalities, Pituitary gland, Hormones

Intracranial Arachnoid Cysts: A quantitative analysis of fluid dynamics and continuous intracystic pressure monitoring
—A new concept of "localized hydrocephalus"—

Shizuo Oi, Yoshiteru Shose, Yasuhiro Okuda, Hiroshi Yamada, Akihiro Ijichi, and Satoshi Matsumoto

Department of Neurosurgery, Kobe University, School of Medicine, Kobe, Japan

The natural history and pathophysiology of intracranial arachnoid cysts are still obscure. The purpose of this paper is to analyze the characteristics of the fluid dynamics of arachnoid cysts by utilizing the quantitative analysis method of metrizamide CT cisternography (CTCG). These results are then compared with those of intracystic pressure dynamics. We discuss the pathophysiology of and the operative indication for intracranial arachnoid cysts.
The patterns of fluid dynamics in arachnoid cysts in the major pathway of CSF circulation are various. It is not possible to classify 3 or 4 types of cyst-CSF circulation patterns, as has been done in many previous reports, with just this quantitative analysis method, namely, CTCG. There was no close correlation between the type of fluid communication and either clinical symptoms or intracystic pressure dynamics.
From these points of view, it was suggested that the operative or therapeutic goal in treating arachnoid cysts is to normalize the pressure dynamics, which are likely to damage the regional brain function with its expansile ballooning pressure in non-communicating cysts or stagnating fluid force in communicating cysts. We hereby propose a new concept of "localized hydrocephalus" with regard to intracranial arachnoid cysts.

(CT Kenkyu 8: 413–420, 1986)

Key words: Arachnoid cyst, Fluid dynamics, Pressure dynamics, Hydrocephalus, Localized hydrocephalus

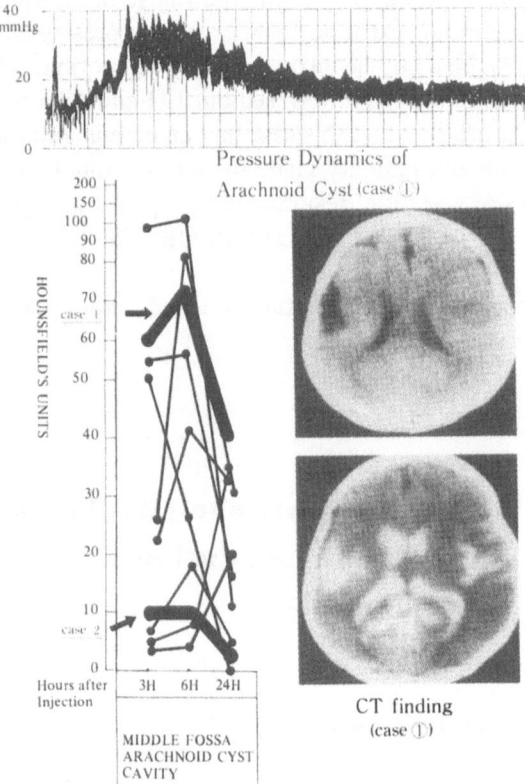

Pressure Dynamics of
Arachnoid Cyst (case ①)

Fluid Dynamics of
Arachnoid Cyst

CT finding
(case ①)

Figure 1. Pressure pattern in arachnoid cyst cavity in a case of "communicating arachnoid cyst." Note remarkable pressure wave and high base line pressure.

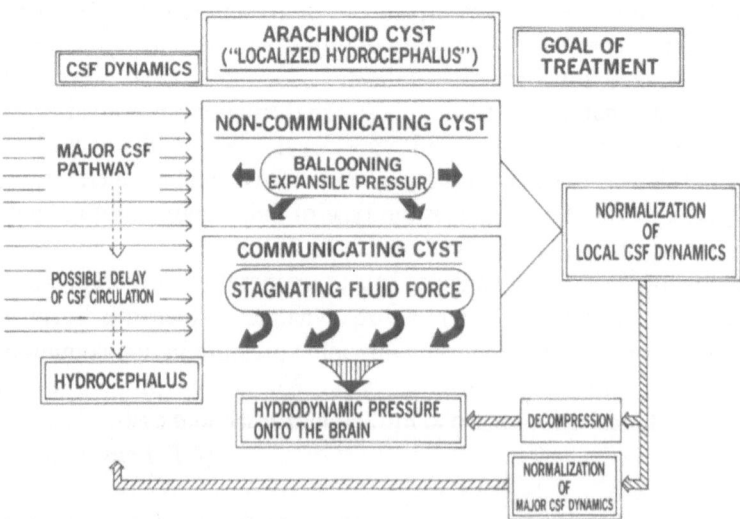

Figure 2. Concepts of arachnoid cyst as "localized hydrocephalus."

Fluid Secretion in Arachnoid Cysts as a Clue to Cerebrospinal Fluid Absorption at the Arachnoid Granulation

K. Gwan Go and Hendrik Jan Houthoff

Departments of Neurosurgery and Pathology, University of Groningen, Groningen, The Netherlands

Although the role of arachnoid villi and arachnoid granulations in the absorption of cerebrospinal fluid (CSF) has been well established, the precise mechanism is still the subject of controversy. An open system of endothelium-lined channels in the arachnoid granulations (occurring in larger animals only) has been indicated by previous observations.[1,2] These open channels are envisaged to constitute a valvular mechanism for the transport of CSF from the subendothelial spaces in the core of the granulation to the sinus lumen. However, other observations[3,4] have indicated an uninterrupted layer of endothelial cells lining arachnoid granulations and arachnoid villi in smaller animals as well, envisaging a closed system, in which vacuoles are formed in the endothelial cytoplasm from invaginations of the subendothelial space, and subsequently empty into the vascular lumen after traversing the endothelial cytoplasm.

Next to these biomechanical mechanisms, the possibility of a biochemical absorptive mechanism has been suggested by the following observations. The cells covering arachnoid granulations showed a morphological similarity to the cells of the subdural neurothelium[5,6] and to the cells lining arachnoid cysts. Arachnoid cysts are cavities filled with a CSF-like fluid, which are seggregated from the normal CSF spaces, and on the basis of the morphology of their lining could be regarded as malformations derived from the subdural neurothelium.[7] By enzyme ultracytochemistry (on the basis of the p-nitrophenylphosphatase reaction) the presence of transport $Na^+K^+ATPase$ could be demonstrated in the plasma membrane of the cells lining arachnoid cysts, as an indication of their secretory capacity.[8] Also in the luminal plasma membrane of endothelial cells lining human arachnoid granulations $Na^+K^+ATPase$ could be demonstrated by enzyme ultracytochemistry, suggesting that in the process of CSF absorption a biochemical transport mechanism may play a role.[9] In support of a biochemical mechanism is the reported effect of dexamethasone, which in perfusion studies of arachnoid villi proved to be capable of reducing the opening pressure.[10]

(J Neurosurg 65: 642–648, 1986)

Key words: CSF absorption, Arachnoid granulation, Arachnoid cyst, Na^+K^+-ATPase ultracytochemistry

References
1) Welch, K., Friedman, V.: Brain, 83: 454–469, 1960.
2) Jayatilaka, A.D.P.: J. Anat., 99: 635–649, 1965.

3) Alksne, J.F., Lovings, E.T.: Arch. Neurol., 27: 371–377, 1972.
4) Shabo, A.L., Maxwell, D.S.: J. Neurosurg., 29: 451–463, 1968.
5) Rascol, M., Izard, I: J. Microscopie, 8: 1017–1030, 1969.
6) Andres, K.H.: Z. Zellforsch., 82: 92–109, 1967.
7) Go, K.G., Houthoff, H.J., *et al.*: Acta Neuropathol., 44: 57–62, 1978.
8) Go, K.G., Houthoff, H.J., *et al.*: J. Neurosurg., 60: 803–813, 1984.
9) Go, K.G., Houthoff, H.J., *et al.*: J. Neurosurg., 65: 642–648, 1986.
10) Love, J.A., Fridén, H., Ekstedt, J.: In: Recent Progress in the Study and Therapy of Brain Edema. Go, K.G., Baethmann, A.(Eds.), Plenum, New York, 589–595, 1984.

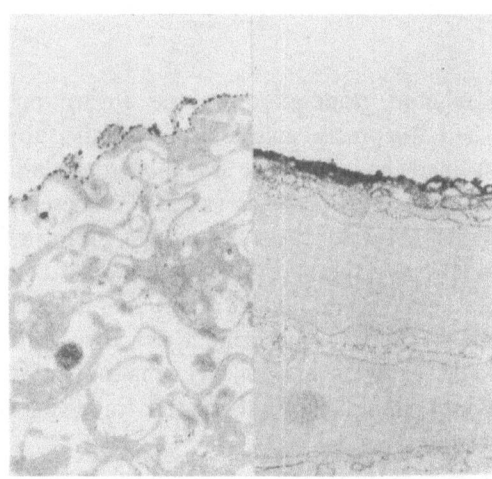

Figure. Enzyme ultracytochemical test for K^+-nitrophenylphosphatase in the lining of an arachnoid cyst (*left*) and arachnoid granulation (*right*). The reaction product, indicating Na^+K^+-ATPase activity, is situated at the apical plasma membrane of the lining cell layer.

Colloid Cysts of the Third Ventricle:
Open operative approach or stereotactic aspiration?

E. Donauer,[1] J. R. Moringlane,[2] and C. B. Ostertag[2]

[1]Department of Neurosurgery, University of Saarland; and [2]Department of Stereotactic Neurosurgery, University of Saarland, Homburg/Saar, FRG

Colloid cysts of the third ventricle can cause hydrocephalus if they grow to the point where they occlude the foramina interventricularia. The operative approach via a craniotomy used to be the common method of treating these lesions. Now, in the era of CT-and MR-scanning, stereotactic aspiration should be preferred as an ideal method of simultaneously, diagnosing and treating colloid cysts. Unlike open surgery, aspiration of colloid masses poses hardly any risk for the patient.

Ten patients, 7 male and 3 female, aged between 14 and 64 years, mean 43 years, were successfully treated by this stereotactic technique. In all cases signs of intermittent increasing brain pressure, as headache, memory disturbance, gait instability and dizziness lead to hospital admission. Two patients showed an intermittent hemihypaesthesia. In 6 cases, shunting treatment of hydrocephalus had been performed beforehand in other hospitals. With gentle aspiration and irrgation stereotactic evacuation of the cysts was possible in every case. The mucous contents can be very viscous. The cannula used for aspiration therefore should be no less than 1.4 mm in inner diameter. After aspitation the cysts were filled with air and contrast medium to radiographically demonstrate the complete removal of the cyst contents. For histological determination a biopsy of the cystwall was performed.

The cysts could be evacuated in all cases without any complications. We did not observe any recurrences of the cysts.

With regard to its safety and the lack of complications and approach-related sideeffects the stereotactic evacuation of colloid cysts of the third ventricle should be regarded as treatment of choice and at the same time as method for establishing the definite histological diagnosis.

(Acta Neurochir 83: 24–30, 1986)

Key words: Colloid cysts, Hydrocephalus, Stereotactic puncture, Third ventricle

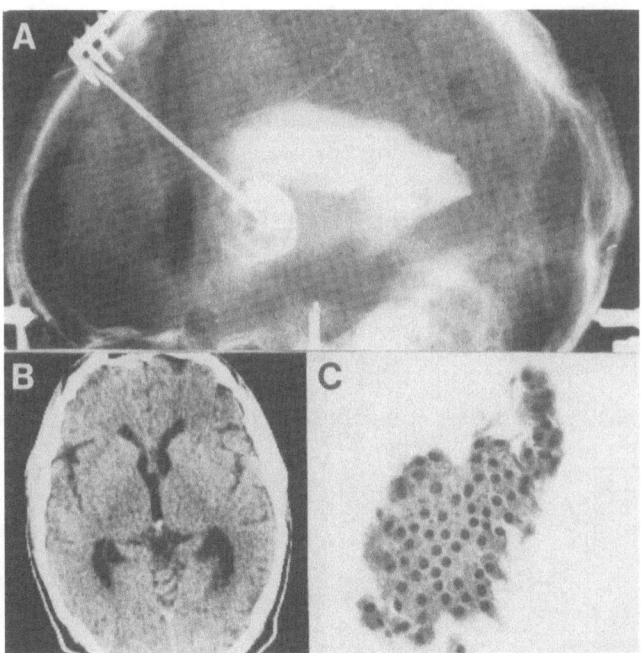

Figure. (A) Lateral view of the ventriculogram shows the cannula in the partially aspirated colloid cyst.
(B) By stereotactic aspiration a colloid cyst has been verified and at the same time evacuated.
(C) A smear preparation of the cyst-wall shows the typical cuboidal epithelium of the colloid cysts.

Demonstration of a Symptomatic Intraventricular Cyst Using Direct Intraventricular Metrizamide Instillation

Rita Jeannette Marie Blom,[1] Norbert Witt,[2] and Edward Stedworthy Johnson[3]

Departments of [1]Radiology, [2]Neurology, and [3]Pathology, University of Alberta Hospitals, Edmonton, Alberta, Canada

A 30-year-old man presented with a "pressure" sensation in the left occipital and frontal regions. For the previous four months he suffered from rage attacks, brief losses of consciousness and occasional numbness of his right side.

A CT scan with intravenous contract (Conray 60–100 ccs) demonstrated a mass lesion of CSF density displacing the left choroid plexus arteriolaterally. The occipital horn was dilated and the margins of the lesion were not distinct. Direct intraventricular instillation through a burr hole of 3 ccs of metrizamide (170 mg/m*l*) outlined the lesion well. The cyst was totally resected at surgery, neuropathological studies were considered sufficient to classify this lesion as a choroid plexus cyst.

Choroid plexus cysts are frequent at autopsy in the lateral ventricles and may represent a degenerative change. These cysts, along with ependymal cysts, epithelial cysts, colloid cysts and even teratogenous cysts are classified by some as neuroepithelial cysts. Since publication of this articles, two other young men have been studied with headaches and similar enhanced CT findings. Their clinical condition was not severe enough to warrant further investigation and treatment.   (AJNR 7: 1093–1095, 1986)

Key words: Metrizamide, Intraventricular, Cyst, Choroid plexus, Neuroepithelial cyst, CT scan

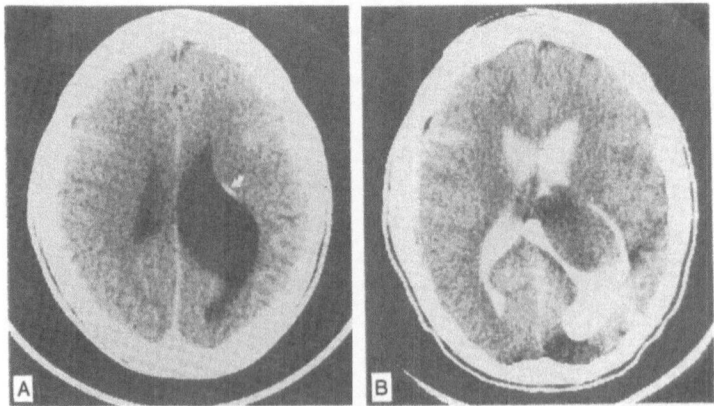

Figure. (A) Axial CT scan after intravenous contrast (Conray). Arrow points to displaced choroid plexus. Cyst walls are not seen.
(B) Axial CT scan after metrizamide instillation. Ellipsoid cyst does not fill with contrast.

Cavum Vergae Cyst as a Cause of Hydrocephalus Almost Forgotten?: Successful causal stereotactic treatment

E. DONAUER, J. R. MORINGLANE, and Chr. B. OSTERTAG

Department of Stereotactic Neurosurgery of the Saarland University, Homburg/Saar, FRG

In 1851 the italian anatomist VERGA first described a cystic formation in the brain midline between the columnae fornicorum in the prolongation of the septum pellucidum. This cystic formation was named cavum vergae (CVC), which was thus distinguished from the cavum septi pellucidi. The cavum vergae usually communicates with the cavum septi pellucidi, but in some cases both are separated by a membrane. CVC are cerebral midline malformations, which usually have no clinical manifestation. In rare cases, however, non-communicating cysts can cause a hydrocephalus by obstruction of the aquaeduct.

Initially, from the 1930th through the 1960th, operative treatment consisted in open cysto-ventriculostomy, *i.e.* establishing a communication between CVC and the ventricles, via a transventricular approach. In the era of CT, symptomatic treatment of the hydrocephalus by ventriculo-cardial or peritoneal shunting is preferred, which inherits all the wellknown complications of shunting treatment. Based on the experience with our cases of

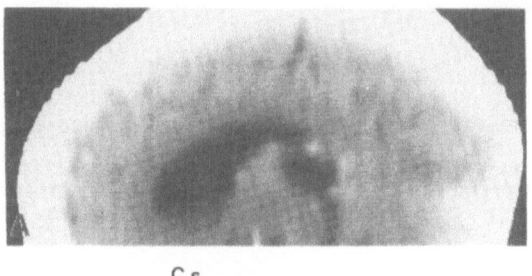

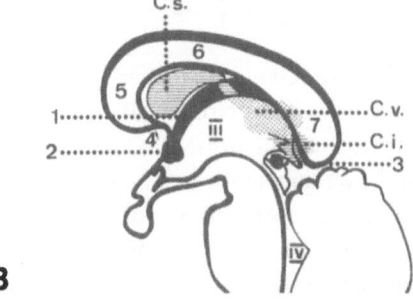

Figure. (A) lateral view in reconstructed CT-image, (B) artit's view: C.s.: cavum septum pellucidi, C.v.: cavum vergae, C.i.: cisterna interventricularis, 1: columna fornicis, 2: commissura anterior, 3: commissura posterior, 4: rastrum corporis callosi, 5: genu corporis callosi, 6: truncus corporis callosi, 7: splenium corporis callosi, III: the third ventricle, IV: the fourth ventricle.

CVC with clinical manifestation, we here propose a definitive causal treatment which can be achieved by draining the cyst contents into the ventricles via a stereotactically introduced catheter.

One male patient (63 years old) and three female patients (11, 22, 36 years old) were referred to our hospital one week, one month, 6 months and 5 years respectively after the onset of symptoms, as were headaches, diplopia, confusion and in a child mental retardation. In these four patients, a relatively small CVC has led to an intermittent occlusive hydrocephalus by compression of the posterior part of the third ventricle and aquaeduct. An increase in intracranial pressure was documented by ICP-monitoring. Other causes of hydrocephalus could not be found. Stereotactic puncture confirmed the cystic nature suggested by the CT-images. During the same session an internal drainage was performed. All patients remained symptomfree during a followup between 6 months and three years.

(Acta Neurochir 83: 12–19, 1986)

Key words: Intracerebral midline cysts, Cavum vergae, Developmental cystic malformations, Hydrocephalus, Stereotactic surgery

Neurofibromatosis with Aqueductal Stenosis and Cavum Septi Pellucidi

Yoji Komatsu,[1] Takao Enomoto,[1] Tadao Nose,[1] Yutaka Maki,[1] and Takayuki Matsuki[2]

[1]Department of Neurosurgery, Institute of Clinical Medicine, University of Tsukuba, Tsukuba;
[2]Department of Neurosurgery, Kensei General Hospital, Ibaraki, Japan

A 10-year-old boy was admitted to Kensei General Hospital with complaints of limitation of eye movement, and gait disturbance. His head circumstance had been about 90 percentile large since the birth. Six months previous to the present admission dysarrthria appeared, and gait disturbance progressed. His head circumstance had been about 90 percentile large since the birth. Six months previous to the present admission dysarrthria appeared, and gait disturbance progressed. His activity decreased, and sometimes he vomited. Three months later, CT scan showed non-communicating hydrocephaly. He was admitted to the hospital. On physical examination, cafe au lait spots were evident.   He also had pretectal syndrome. The first ventricular peritoneal shunt operation was carried out using low pressure system without antisiphon device. Over drainage occurred, and then subdural hematoma appeared. The shunt system was changed to medium pressure. This time intracranial pressure increased, and his consciousness deteriorated. Low pressure with antisiphon device was used at the third operation. His condition returned to the previous state, but subdural effusion reappeared. Then he was referred to our hospital for further treatment. We inserted him two shunt systems in; VP shunt using low pressure valve with antisiphon, and subdural space peritoneal shunt using low pressure tube only. His neurological state improved, and CT also returned to normal one. It is thought that the gliosis around the aqueduct produces non-communicating hydrocephalus in neurofibromatosis patients. Only 10 cases were reported to have pathologically proven aqueductal stenosis. In about half of the patients with neurofibromatosis, the dilatation of the ventricles was observed, and this was thought to be due to the effect of cerebrovascular disease of neurofibromatosis. In cases with cranio-cerebral disproportion like our case, shunt operation sometimes causes trouble. The simultaneous double shunting with different pressure resistance can be benefit in such a case.

(*Shoni no Noshinkei* 11: 325–330, 1986)

Key words: Neurofibromatosis, Hydrocephalus, Aqueductal stenosis, Macrocranium, Cavum septi pellucidi

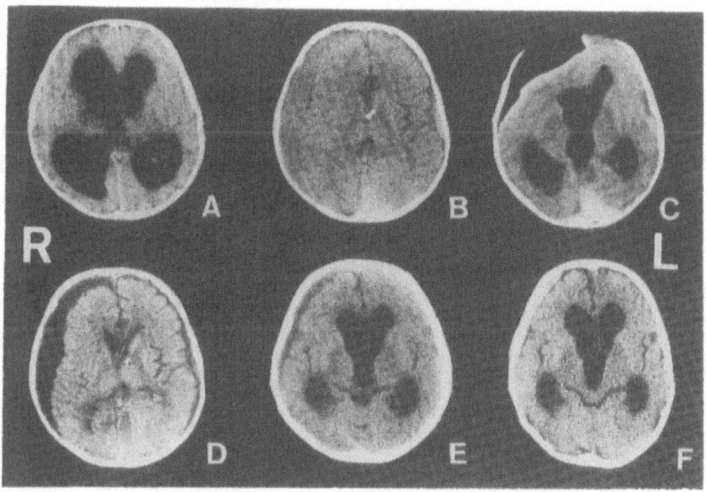

Figure. CT scans (**A**) On the admission to the previous hospital. (**B**) After the first ventricle peritoneal shunt operation. (**C**) After the hematoma removal. (**D**) After the third shunt operation. (**E**) On the admission to our hospital. (**F**) After the ventricle peritoneal shunt, and the subdural space peritoneal shunt operation.

Hydrocephalus, Lissencephaly, Ocular Abnormalities and Congenital Muscular Dystrophy:
A Warburg syndrome variant?

L. Pavone, F. Gullotta, S. Grasso, and C. Vannucchi

Institut für Neuropathologie der Universität Münster, FRG

The authors describe a family in whom three members suffered from congenital hydrocephalus and ocular abnormalities. One of these childpatient showed along with these symptoms congenital muscular dystrophy. In this child, autopsy disclosed severe cerebral malformations consisting of lissencephaly, arhinencephaly, stenosis of aqueduct, Dandy-Walker cyst and cerebellar micropolygyria. The mode of transmission, the eyes abnormalities and the neuropathological findings of this family resemble the clinical and pathological aspects of Warburg syndrome (hydrocephalus, microphthalmia and congenital retinal nonattachment). However, the presence of congenital muscle dystrophy in one of these children suggests some links with Fukuyama's congenital muscular dystrophy and/or with so-called brain-eye-muscle disease of Santavuori. These three syndromes are shortly discussed.

Summarized in *Table* a few similar literature cases presenting these main symptoms and published under different eponyms-F-CMD; muscle-eye-brain disease Santavuori's; Walker-

Table. Summary of reported cases presenting "congenital cerebro-ocular myopathy syndrome"

1. Fukuyama *et al.* 1981: case 3	male, 9 months
2. Fukuyama *et al.* 1981: case 11	female, 3 months
3. Fukuyama *et al.* 1981: case 12	female, 2 years
4. Krijgsman *et al.* 1980	male, 4 months
5. Dambska *et al.* 1982: 1st case (brother of 2 and 3)	male, sev. months
6. Dambska *et al.* 1982: 2nd case	female, 4 months
7. Dambska *et al.* 1982: 3rd case	male, stillborn
8. Korinthenberg *et al.* 1984	female, 9 months
9. Towfighi *et al.* 1984: 1st case	male, 4 months
10. Towfighi *et al.* 1984: 2nd case (brother of 1)	male, 12 months
11. Towfighi *et al.* 1984: 3rd case	male, 5 months
12. Towfighi *et al.* 1984: 4th case (sister of 3)	female, 5 months
13. Towfighi *et al.* 1984: 5th case	female, 10 months
14. Towfighi *et al.* 1984: 6th case	male, 44 gest. weeks
15. Towfighi *et al.* 1984: 7th case (brother of 6)	male, 6 days
16. Williams *et al.* 1984: 3rd case	female, 15 months
17. Present case	male, 13 months

Warburg syndrome. These cases might represent a clinical variant of the Warburg syndrome or, on the other side, the most severe form of a congenital complex syndrome involving brain, muscle and eyes, for which the definition "Congenital Cerebro-Ocular-Myopathy syndrome (CoCOM syndrome)" is proposed. In author's opinion, the generical term syndrome is more appropriate for this clinical-morphological picture, instead of dysplasia as suggested by Towfighi et al. 1984. It is of course possible that we are dealing with three different nosological entities. But it cannot a priori be excluded that the three syndromes of Warburg, Fukuyama and Santavuori may represent three variants of the one and same disease, which can affect only brain and eyes (Warburg) or muscle and brain (Fukuyama) or all three organs, but in milder form (Santavuori).

Further clinical and morphological studies are needed to detect the cause of these syndromes, which are probably more common as suspected.

(Neuropediatrics 17: 206–211, 1986)

Key words: Warburg syndrome, Lissencephaly, Congenital muscular dystrophy

Aneurysm of the Vein of Galen in an Infant: Case report

Shinji Sugimoto,[1] Terufumi Itoh,[2] Hiroshi Abe,[1] Yoku Nakagawa,[1] Fumio Itoh,[1] Kohei Echizenya,[1] and Mitsuyuki Koiwa[3]

[1,2,3]Department of Neurosurgery, Hokkaido University School of Medicine, Sapporo, Japan; Present address: [2]Nikko Memorial Hospital and [3]Kashiwaba Neurosurgical Hospital

A case of an aneurysm of the vein of Galen treated by a successful direct surgical procedure during the infancy is presented together with five year's follow-up observation.

This female child who had suffered from heart failure in the neonatal period was admitted to our hospital at the age of eight month because of psychomotor retardation and seizures. At that time, CT scan revealed hydrocephalus, periventricular calcified areas and a mass lesion in the posterior aspect of the third ventricle. Subsequent cerebral angiography confirmed the diagnosis of an aneurysm of the vein of Galen. After the bilateral parieto-occipital craniotomy, interhemispheric approach to the lesion was performed through the right and left sides of the falx. This method provided a good exposure of the aneurysm to clip the feeding arteries successfully. Postoperative CT scans demonstrated the thrombosed and collapsed aneurysm.

However, the child showed marked developmental disturbance even at the time of five years after the surgical treatment. It was speculated that the poor functional prognosis of this patient was due to wide-spread brain damages which had been suspected from preoperative CT findings.

From the experience of this case, we want to emphasize the need for early diagnosis and treatment during the infancy to obtain better functional prognosis in such a potentially lethal disease.   (*Shoni no Noshinkei* 11: 15–22, 1986)

Key words: Aneurysm of the vein of Galen, Hydrocephalus, Arteropvenous malformation

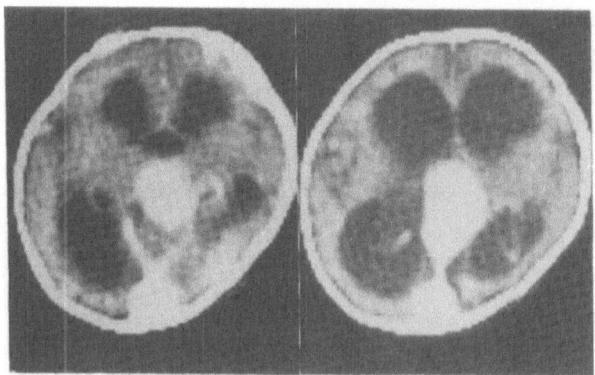

Figure.   Postoenhancement CT scans.
There is a mass (aneurysm) which showed marked homogenous enhancement in the posterior aspect of the third ventricle.
Hydrocephalus and periventricular calcified foci are also noted.

Evaluation of Apparently Hydrocephalic CT Findings in Fukuyama Type Congenital Muscular Dystrophy with RI Cisternography and Serial CT Scannings

Yukio Fukuyama,[1] Youich Mitsuishi,[1] Makiko Osawa,[1] Keiko Shishikura,[1] Atsushi Kohno,[2] and Masako Maki[2]

Department of [1]Pediatrics and [2]Radiology, Tokyo Women's Medical College, Tokyo, Japan

Fukuyama type congenital muscular dystrophy (FCMD) which was first described by Fukuyama *et al.* is recognized as a well-established clinical entity, and is characterized by accompanying CNS symptoms (intellectual impairment, convulsion) and pathological abnormalities of the CNS (ventricular dilatation, micro-polygyria, etc.). CT scan usually shows mild to moderate ventricular dilatation accompanied by low density area (LDA) in periventricular white matter which resembles periventricular lucency in hydrocephalus.

These findings of CT scan suggested possibility of involvement of hydrocephalic process in the pathogenesis of brain dysplasia in this condition. In addition, a few FCMD cases with hypertensive hydrocephalus had been reported. Furthermore, some cases of Walker-Warburg syndrome were revealed to have a combination of brain, eye and muscle abnormalities. Therefore, the present study was undertaken to determine whether the hydrocephalic state is present or not in FCMD cases. RI cisternography was performed in 10 cases of typical FCMD, and CT scans were serially carried out in 14 cases of FCMD including 2 atypical cases.

Results: In RI cisternography, pathological ventricular stasis was demonstrated in one case, early ventricular reflux in 8 cases of the rest, clearance delay in all cases and laterality without asymmetry in CT scan in 2 cases. In serial CT scan examinations, both ventricular dilatation and LDA in periventricular white matter decreased in degree with increasing age in all cases but 2. An exceptional case was present which had pathological ventricular stasis in RI citsternography and slowly progressive ventricular dilatation on CT scan, but he had no signs of ICP elevation. Although results of RI cisternography suggest an abnormality in CSF dynamics, but its significance is difficult to determine. Spontaneous improvement of CT scan findings with age suggests an absence of active hydrocephalic process in this disease.

(Annual Report of the Research Committee of "Hydrocephalus," The Ministry of Health and Welfare of Japan, 1986: 111–118, 1987)

Key words: Fukuyama type congenital muscular dystrophy, CT scan, RI cisternography, Hydrocephalus

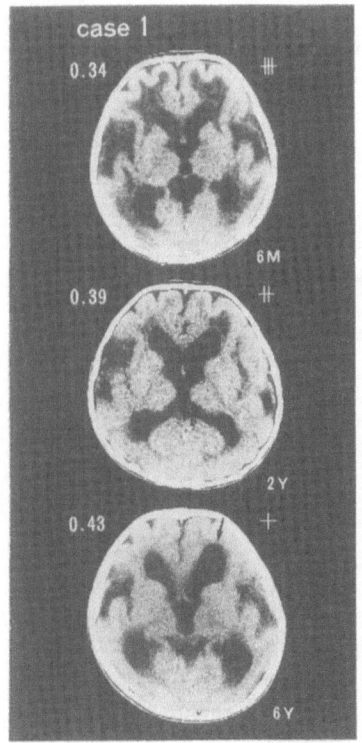

Figure. Serial CT scans in Case 1, +, ++, +++ denote white matter lucency of mild, moderate and severe degrees respectively. The numbers on the left side of the Figure indicate Evans' ratios.

Infantile Choroid Plexus Papilloma

Hirokazu Kawano,[1] Minoru Hayashi,[1] Toshihiko Kubota,[1] Akira Ishikura,[2] Hidenori Kobayashi,[1] and Tetsuro Tsuji[1]

[1]Department of Neurosurgery, Fukui Medical School, Fukui; [2]Department of Neurosurgery, National Kanazawa Hospital, Kanazawa, Japan

Papilloma of the choroid plexus which causes hydrocephalus is an unusual but more common in childhood and curable by surgical treatment. While the results of the treatment for this tumor in early infants have not been satisfactory. Treatment of the hydrocephalus which is complicated with papilloma is very important for the post operative prognosis. This report describes the histogenesis, the diagnosis and the treatment of this tumor on the basis of authors experiences through three cases which were successfully treated with surgery. Case 1, a 10-month-old boy, had an enlarged skull at birth and was brought to our clinic because of frequent vomiting since 6 months old. Case 2, an 8-month-old girl, was referred to our clinic because of retarded growth and recurrent vomiting since 2 months old. Case 3, a 6-month-old boy, developed a large head at 2 months old and had fallen into shock state at 3 months old. Case 1 and 2 have grown normally after removal of the tumor and ventriculoperitoneal shunt. On the other hand case 3 has shown a psychomotor retardation because of poorly controlled hydrocephalus.   (*Shoni no Noshinkei* 11: 193–198, 1986)

Key words: Choroid plexus papilloma, Early infants, Hydrocephalus, V-P shunt

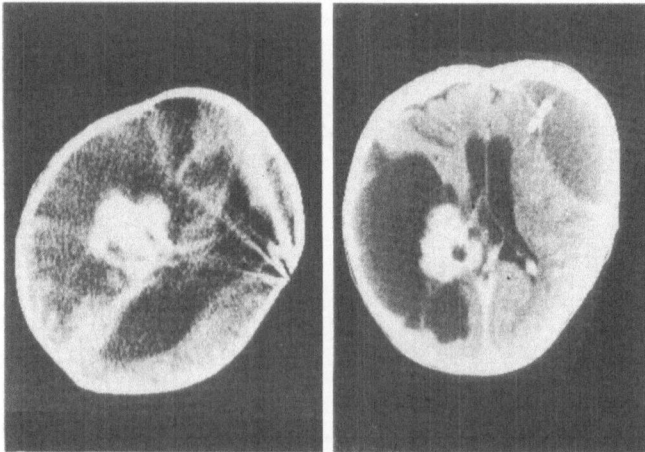

Figure. CT scans with contrat infusion (Case 3) show a high density area in the right lateral ventricle with hydrocephalus (*left*) and left subdural hematoma after V-P shunt (*right*).

Meningioma in the Anterior III Ventricle in a Child

Han-Jung CHEN,[1] Chun-Chung LUI,[2] and Leung CHEN[3]

[1]Division of Neurosurgery, Department of Surgery, [2]Department of Radiology, and [3]Department of Pathology, Chang Gung Memorial Hospital, Kaohsiung Medical Center, Kaohsiung, Taiwan, ROC

The occurrence of meningiomas in the III ventricle is very rare. Only 37 cases have been reported. There appears to be a higher incidence of this location in children than in adults. A case is described of meningioma in the anterior part of the III ventricle in a 14-year-old girl. The mass was successfully removed through a transcallosal approach. Cerebral angiogram showed the feeder was from the posterior medial choroidal artery. The draining vein was the internal cerebral vein.
Histopathological examination showed whorl formation in this meningioma.

(Child's Nerv Syst 2: 160–161, 1986)

Key words: Meningioma, III ventricle, Hydrocephalus

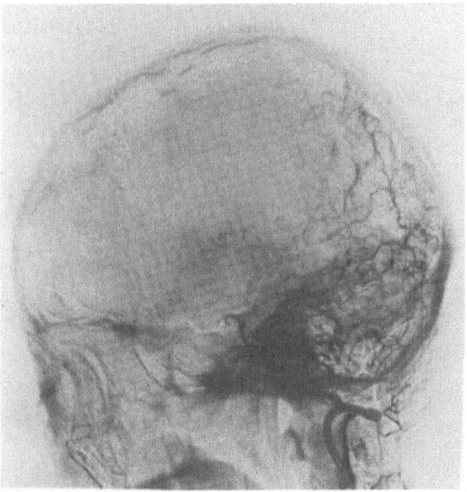

Figure. Vertebral angiogram showing the feeder from the posterior medial choroidal artery, and tumor vessels.

A Case of Pineocytoma Presenting with Symptoms like Normal Pressure Hydrocephalus

Ichiro Sayama,[1] Nobuyuki Yasui,[1] Hitoshi Fukasawa,[2] Masahito Nemoto,[1] and Hidenori Ohta[1]

Departments of [1]Surgical Neurology and [2]Pathology, Research Institute for Brain and Blood Vessels-AKITA, Akita, Japan

A pineocytoma in an old man, whose initial symptoms resembled a normal pressure hydrocephalus, is reported. This 67-year-old man gradually became uncommunicative and difficult to walk alone in three months. Just before visiting our clinic, his family also noticed his nocturnal urinary incontinence. CT scan on admission disclosed tumor in the posterior wall of the third ventricle, and subsequent hydrocephalus. This oval, isodense tumor was homogeneously enhanced after the injection of contrast medium on CT scan.

The vertebral angiography showed a mass in the pineal region with no vascular staining. Ventricular drainage, the opening pressure of which was 100 mmH$_2$O, could not offer cytological verfication of the tumor.

By the infratentorial supracerebeller approach, the tumor was successfully extirpated, and the post-operative course was uneventful.

The microscopic study revealed the nature of this tumor to be well compatible with that of a pineocytoma.   (*Noshinkeigeka* 14: 789–794, 1986)

Key words: Pineocytoma, Normal pressure hydrocephalus, Pathological study, Treatment

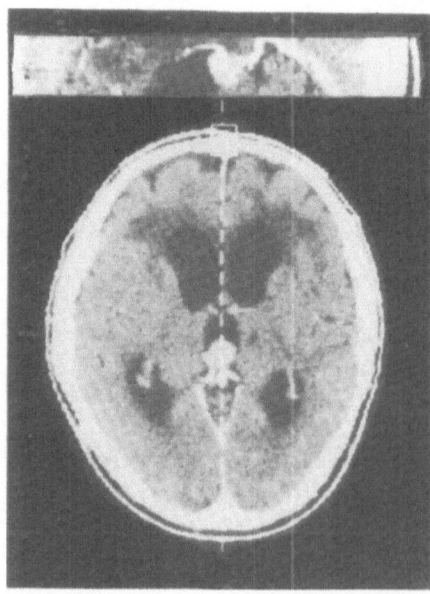

Figure. CT scan findings on admission. Enhanced CT. The upper image shows the reconstructive view on the mid-sagittal plane indicated by the dotted line. The posterior half of the third ventricle is occupied by the spherical mass which is homogeneously stained with contrast media. Subsequently a hydrocephalus with periventricular lucency is seen. The old lacune on the left thalamus is also noted.

Management of Posthemorrhagic Hydrocephalus in the Preterm Infant

Mujahid Anwar, Aiden J. Doyle, Shilpa Kadam, I. Mark Hiatt, and Thomas Hegyi

Departments of Pediatrics and Neurosurgery, University of Medicine and Dentistry of New Jersey, Robert Wood Johnson Medical School, New Brunswick, NJ, USA

Hydrocephalus is a common sequel to a moderate or large intraventricular hemorrhage (IVH) in preterm infants. Progressive ventricular dilation and increased intracranial pressure usually occur within two to three weeks of age. At this time, these infants are still small and suffer from multiple medical problems which make them poor risks for surgical procedures. We studied the use of a subcutaneous ventricular catheter reservoir in 19 preterm infants with posthemorrhagic hydrocephalus. At the time of diagnosis, a ventriculoperitoneal shunt could not be inserted because of medical complications, small size or hemorrhage ventricular fluid. We inserted the reservoir under local anesthesia, supplemented with narcotics in small sick infants, or under general anesthesia in bigger medically stable infants. We aspirated the reservoir daily removing 8–10 ml of fluid. We repeated the procedure if the fontanelle became full and tense 8–12 hours after the first reservoir aspiration. We inserted the reservoir at 29 ± 9 days of postnatal age and 1217 ± 414 grams body weight.
We maintained the reservoir in place for 51 ± 29 days. We removed 527 ± 421 ml of fluid by performing 57 ± 42 reservoir aspirations. All infants tolerated the procedure well. Only two infants developed infection despite multiple reservoir aspirations. One infant expired due to unrelated causes. Ten infants developed hyponatremia requiring sodium supplementation. Two infants developed local fluid leak which was controlled with more frequent reservoir aspirations. Three infants did not require a permanent shunt. We inserted a ventriculo-peritoneal shunt in 15 infants prior to discharge from the newborn nursery at 3 to 4 months of age. We conclude that ventricular catheter reservoir is a safe and effective palliative procedure in the management of posthemorrhagic hydrocephalus in small preterm infants.

(J Pediatr Surg 21: 334–337, 1986)

Key words: Hydrocephalus, Intraventricular hemorrhage, Ventricular catheter reservoir

Ventricular Septa in the Neonatal Age Group:
Diagnosis and considerations of etiology

Dieter SCHELLINGER,[1] Edward G. GRANT,[1] Herbert J. MANZ,[2] Nicholas PATRONAS,[1] and Ronald H. USCINSKI[3]

[1]Department of Radiology, [2]Department of Pathology, [3]Department of Surgery, Georgetown University Medical Center, Washington, D.C., USA

In this report, twenty-four patients with ventricular septa are discussed. Seventeen patients had neonatally acquired septa and seven exhibited septations at birth (congenital septa). Among the acquired septa, there were true intraventricular septa and septa which originated outside the ventricles but later become part of the ventricular system (pseudosepta). Pseudosepta originate in necrotic, cavitating periventricular white matter that, in temporal sequence, becomes ventricularized. Serial use of cranial ultrasonography provided important information regarding the pathological mechanisms which governed the development of septa. Intraventricular hemorrhage and infection are the major causes of true intraventricular septa while periventricular leukomalacia serves as primary cause of pseudosepta. Sonography is the diagnostic method of choice. Septa are associated with a high incidence (62%) of shunt failure.   (AJNR 7: 1065–1071, 1986)

Key words: Pediatric hydrocephalus, Brain, Septa, Pseudosepta, Shunt failure, Cranial sonography, Intraventricular hemorrhage, Ventriculitis

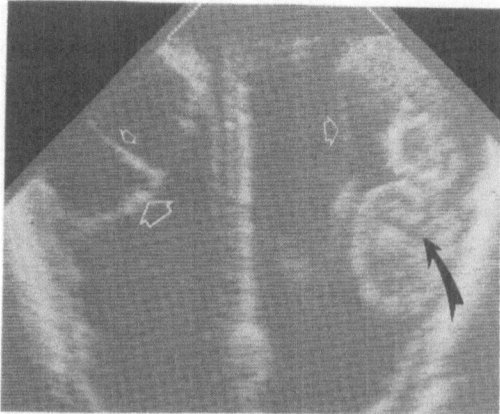

Figure. Premature infant who developed intraventricular hemorrhage and periventricular leukomalacia on 8th day of life.
Periventricular cysts appeared on 15th day of life and pseudosepta emerged on 30th day of life.
Axial sonogram, showing large lateral ventricles.
Pseudosepta are seen in both ventricles (*open arrows*). A large blood clot is contained within one of the ventricles (*large black arrow*).

Destructive Hydrocephalus: A proposed new category

Saburo Nakamura and Takashi Tsubokawa

Department of Neurological Surgery, Nihon University School of Medicine, Tokyo, Japan

Hydrocephalus occurring in region of the brain that have suffered destructive changes from a cause other than that of the hydrocephalus is proposed as a new category ("destructive hydrocephalus"). A case with hydrocephalus subsequent to neonatal intraventricular and intracerebral hemorrhage is reported to belong in such category of hydrocephalus.

The patient was delivered after 26 weeks and 5 days of gestation. Computed tomography showed marked dilation of the left lateral ventricle with high density areas in both lateral ventricle, left hemisphere, and subarachnoid spaces on the left side. Bulging of the anterior fontanelle and vomiting occurred on day 29, and head circumference increased rapidly to day 39. On day 139, the patient was transferred to our department with enlarging lateral ventricles. Hydrocephalus was diagnosed as obstructive, secondary to subarachnoid hemorrhage. However, the lateral ventricle in the hemisphere in which the intracerebral hemorrhage occurred dilated much more than that in the contralateral hemisphere. Ventriculoperitoneal shunt was performed at the age of 153 days. The postoperative convalescence was uneventful. CT scan after surgery revealed irregular dilatation of the ventricle remained. Right hemiplegia and psychomotor developmental delay were noticed even at the age of 2 years.

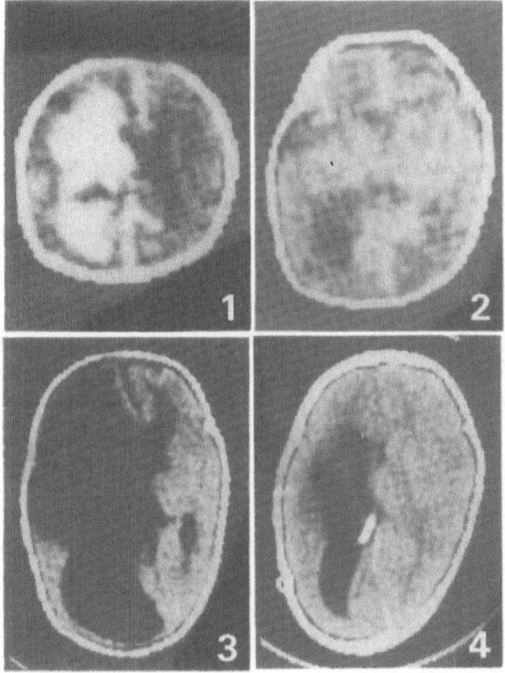

Figure 1. Initial plain CT scans 1 day after birth revealing a large intracerebral hemorrhage in the left hemisphere, with intraventricular and subarachnoid hemorrhage.

Figure 2. CT scan on day 24 revealing a lowered density of the hematoma.

Figure 3. Plain CT scan on day 144, revealing an extremely dilated left lateral ventricle.

Figure 4. The CT scan 18 months after shunt operation reveals thickening of the cerebral mantle of the left hemisphere.

"Destructive hydrocephalus" is to be distinguished from hydrocephalus with dilated ventricles due to simply to increased intraventricular pressure. In this hydrocephalus dilatation of the ventricles occurs irregularly and rapidly, leading to secondary cerebral destruction. Therefore, treatment to prevent the progressive cerebral damage is required immediately.   (Child's Nerv Syst 2: 101–104, 1986)

Key words: Hydrocephalus, Intraventricular hemorrhage, Intracerebral hemorrhage, Neonate

Lysis of Intraventricular Blood Clot with Urokinase in a Canine Model: Part 2

Dachling Pang, Robert J. Sclabassi, and Joseph A. Horton

Children's Hospital of Pittsburgh, Pittsburgh, PA, USA

It was determined from in vitro experiments that the minimal dose of urokinase required to lyse 10 m*l* of clotted canine blood within a closed space must exceed 10,000 IU. We empirically doubled this minimum effective dose and tested the in vivo safety of injecting 20,000 IU of urokinase every 12 hours for 4 days into the ventricles of six adult mongrel dogs through an implanted catheter-reservoir system. The animals were monitored carefully for local and systemic bleeding by neurological and clinical examination, hematological tests reflecting systemic fibrinolytic status, serial computed tomography, and postmortem histological examinations of the brain, meninges, and peripheral organs. It was found that this intraventricular dose regimen of urokinase did not cause intracranial hemorrhage even though the dogs had recent brain wounds related to transcerebral ventricular catheterization. Mild activation of systemic fibrinolysis, implying passage of the enzyme from ventricle to blood, occurred 4 to 6 hours after each intraventricular injection, but no systemic hemorrhages were seen. This dose regimen also did not cause acute or chronic inflammatory changes in the brain or meninges and did not disturb cerebrospinal fluid circulation.
                                      (Neurosurgery 19: 547–552, 1986)

Key words: Dosage determination, Intraventicular urokinase, Periventricular hemorrhage, Safety study, Systemic plasminogen activation

Use of Intrathecal Hyaluronidase in the Management of Tuberculous Meningitis with Hydrocephalus

S. N. BHAGWATI and Koshy GEORGE

Department of Neurosurgery, Grant Medical College and J. J. Group of Hospitals and Medical Research Centre, Bombay Hospital, Bombay, India

A fair number of persons suffering from tuberculous meningitis develop hydrocephalus and raised intracranial pressure due to impairment of CSF circulation as a result of formation of thick basal exudate. Intrathecal hyaluronidase was used in a preliminary study of nine cases with the hope that it would dissolve the exudate, reestablish CSF circulation and potentiate the action of antituberculous drugs. This was followed by a randomised trial in which five cases were treated with intrathecal hyaluronidase while six were treated with ventriculo peritoneal shunt insertion.

No untoward reaction was noted with the use of intrathecal hyaluronidase. Level of consciousness progressively improved in all but 1 of a total of 14 patients (9 of preliminary study and 5 of randomised study) until the 5th or 6th injection of hyaluronidase. Spasticity

Table. Results in terms of specific neurological deficit

		Prelimi-nary Study	Trial	
			Hyaluroni-dase	Shunt
Vision	improved	1/4	—	3/3
	static	2/4	1/1	—
	deteriorated	1/4	—	—
Hemi-paresis	improved	—	2/3	1/3
	static	1/1	1/3	2/3

Overall Results

	Preliminary Study (9 patients)	Trial	
		Hyaluromi-dase (5 patients)	Shunt (6 patients)
good	1	1	2
fair	3	3	1
unchanged	1	1	2
failure	2*	—	—
died	2	—	1

* Both subsequently improved after shunt insertion.

was also reduced in these patients. However, improvement in specific neurological deficit such as vision and hemiparesis was not encouraging. Of five patients with impaired vision, vision improved in one, deteriorated in one and remained static in three. Of four patients with hemiparesis, two showed improvement and two remained static. There were two distinct therapy failures who improved after shunt insertion; vision and sensorium that were deteriorating, improved in both of them thereafter. There were two deaths.

The results for six shunted patients were better. Even patients in Grade IV and V (semicomatose and comatose) showed significant improvement in sensorium; vision improved in all three and hemiparesis improved in one of three, being static in the other two. One patient died after initial improvement.

Overall functional usefulness with normal mentation and regression of neurological deficit like visual impairment and hemiparesis were seen more frequently in the shunted group than in those receiving hyaluronidase. Whereas the shunted group showed a good response in 33% of the patients, only 14% of the hyaluronidase group showed a good response.

(Child's Nerv Syst 2: 20–25, 1986)

Key words: Tuberculous meningitis, Hydrocephalus, Hyaluronidase, Intrathecal hyaluronidase, Intracranial arachnoiditis

Ventriculostomy-related Infections: An epidemiological study

E. Stenager,[1] P. Gerner-Smidt,[2] and C. Kock-Jensen[1]

[1]Department of Neurosurgery, [2]Department of Clinical Microbiology, Odense University Hospital, Odense, Denmark

Previous studies has documented infections related to ventriculostomy when used as a technique for monitoring intracranial pressure and for temporarilly draining cerebrospinal fluid (CSF). Therefore we designed a prospective study including 87 insertions of external ventricular drainage (EVD) in 85 consecutively admitted patients to reveal factors which increased the risk of infection in patients submitted to ventriculostomy.

Extensive information was continously collected at a specific record. Aseptic technique was used when any manipulations of the EVD was carried out. Insertion of the EVD was performed in the theater. CSF samples were cultured at the insertion and removal of the EVD and when patients had fever without any obvious cause or when ventricular infection was suspected clinically.

A diagnosis of probable ventricular infection (PVI) was made when 1) one culture showed ≥ 100 colony forming units (c.f.u.)/0.1 ml CSF or 2) growth of < 100 c.f.u./0.1 ml in 2 or more cultures.

According to our definitions 15 patients (17.2%) were accepted as having PVI. The diagnosis of PVI-patients was subarachnoid haemorrhage (6), tumor (5), hydrocephalus (1) and trauma (3). The bacteriological findings were dominated by low-pathogenic Grampositive cocci (12). The rest were alpha-haemolytic Streptococcus (1), Streptococcus faecalis (1), xanthomas species (1) and acinetobacter calcoaceticus Biotype lwoffi (1).

Table shows the analysis of possible risk factors for the development of PVI. There was no association between the mean duration of the EVD placement and infection nor between the age of the patient and PVI.

We concluded that 1) manipulations with the EVD can be done without increasing the rate of infection as long as strict aseptic technique is used 2) patient with intraventricular haemorrhage in need of EVD are at increased risk of infection and should be monitored bacteriologically regarly. Considering point 1) and 2) our study points to the fact that EVD could be left in place for as long as required.   (Acta Neurochir (Wien) 83: 20–23, 1986)

Key words: Ventriculostomy, Infection, Subarachnoid haemorrhage

Table. Analysis of possible risk factors for EVD related infections

No. of patients with	PVI		no PVI		
Risk factor	Factor present	Factor not present	Factor present	Factor not present	P-value* present
Blood in the CSF+	10	5	26	46	0.029
Duration of EVD placement 11 days	14	1	48	24	0.031
Manipulation more than 5 times	9	6	33	39	0.24
Male sex	12	3	36	36	0.030
Ward A	9	6	40	32	0.49
Antibiotics given from time of insertion of EVD	1	14	9	63	0.43
Complicated skull fracture	1	14	3	69	0.53

* Fischer's exact test.
+ Blood in the CSF was defined as macroscopically visible blood in the CSF, for more than two days.

Normal Pressure Hydrocephalus after Subarachnoid Hemorrhage: With regard to pathogenesis and factors influencing the efficacy of shunt surgery

Koichi KITAMI, Akifumi SUZUKI, Hiromu HADEISHI, Hiromi NISHIMURA, and Nobuyuki YASUI

Department of Surgical Neurology, The Research Institute for Brain and Blood Vessels-AKITA, Akita, Japan

Twenty-four adult cases of suspected normal pressure hydrocephalus (NPH) after subarachnoid hemorrhage (SAH) were investigated clinically from the aspect of predicting the efficacy of the shunting procedure. They consisted of 13 men and 11 women, with the mean age of 55-y-o. In addition to checking neurological signs, pre- and postoperative CT scans, RI (or CT) cisternography and bolus infusion test were performed in each of them. Shunt surgery was done, all of which ventriculoperitoneal shunt, in 17 patients. They were divided into three groups, namely, shunt effective group (A), neurologically unchanged group after surgery (B) and worsened group (C). The A group had 8 cases, B had 8 also and C contained only one. Effectiveness of shunt procedure was measured by an improvement in the activity of daily life (ADL). Compared with group B, group A tended to have more cases of delayed onset of NPH (mean days of 112 from SAH attack in group A while 55 days in group B),

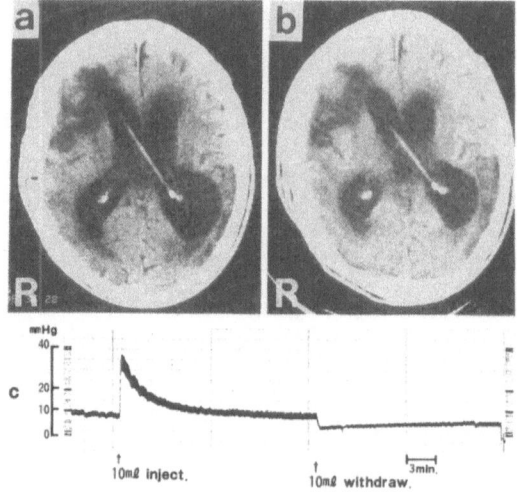

Figure. A case among shunt effective group. (**a**) Immediately after the shunt procedure. The shunt tube was ligated for the infusion test. (**b**) Days after the opening of shunt tube. The ventricular size was becoming small. (**c**) Row data recorded at infusion test.

cases with "trias" (3 against 0) and moderate ventricular dilatation with periventricular lucency (8 against 2). The finding of delayed clearance in cisternogram did not make an accurate judgement in the efficacy of shunt surgery. By using the bolus method of infusion test, the true cause of shunt non-effective ventricular dilatation was suggested to the disturbance of cerebral blood circulation due to elevation of intracranial venous outflow resistance. This suggestion was elicited by the analysis of pressure response curve gained from the bolus injection, in which group A cases mainly reached the baseline pressure within 22 minutes, but on the contrary group B showed more than 22 minutes as a rule. The infusion test also suggested the relatively high cerebrospinal fluid (CSF) productive rate in the shunt effective group. Cases with markedly enlarged ventricle seemed to have stagnated CSF circulation which interrupted the clinical improvement. Shunting procedures were again suggested a good therapeutic method for such cases, if these had worked well in low CSF pressure.   (*No to Shinkei* 38: 781–788, 1986)

Key words: Normal pressure hydrocephalus, CSF shunt, Infusion test

Cerebrovascular Disorders and Dilatation of the Lateral Ventricle

Eiichi OTOMO

Yokufukai Geriatric Hospital, Tokyo, Japan

The relation between cerebrovascular disorders and the volume of the lateral ventricle was studied in 330 consecutive autopsy cases in the Yokufukai Geriatric Hospital.

From these cases, cerebrovascular disorder cases without dementia and clinical episode (39 cases, average age 84.8±6.5 years old) and cases with clinical episode (42 but without dementia average age 84.3±7.3 years old) were selected.

The larger volume of the right lateral ventricle was found in 55% of cases with more severe pathological changes in right hemisphere and this figure was significantly bigger than 9.6%, the ratio of larger right lateral ventricle in 157 subjects with no dementia nor cerebrovascular disorders ($p < 0.01$).

The larger volume of the left lateral ventricle was found in 78.9% cases with more severe pathological changes in the left hemisphere, and this figure was significantly bigger than 48.4%, the ratio which was recognized in 157 cases with no dementia nor cerebrovascular disorders ($p < 0.05$). Similar analysis was conducted in subjects with clinical episode of cerebrovascular disorders. The larger volume of the right lateral ventricle was recognized in 61.9% of cases with more severe pathological changes in the right hemisphere, while the larger volume of the left lateral ventricle was noted in 76.2% of cases with more severe pathological changes in the left hemisphere.

These results suggest that small vascular pathology influences on the volume of the lateral ventricle.

These findings may indicate that vascular pathology is an important factor in dilatation of the lateral ventricle in normal pressure hydrocephalus.

(Annual Report of the Research Committee of "Hydrocephalus," The Ministry of Health and Welfare of Japan, 1986: 175, 1987)

Key words: Lateral ventricle, Cerebrovascular disorders, Ventricle

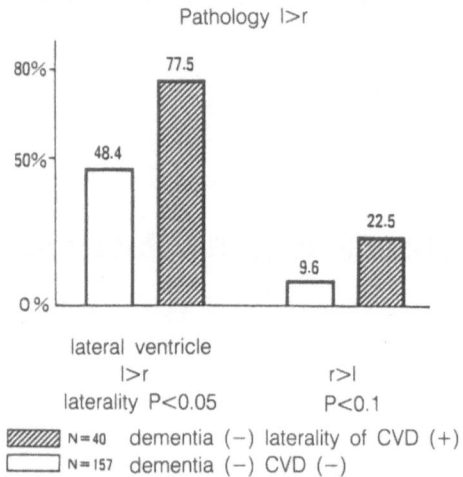

Figure. The lateral ventricle of the side with more obvious vascular pathology is bigger than that of the side with less vascular pathology.

Non-tumoural Aqueduct Stenosis and Normal Pressure Hydrocephalus in the Elderly

Jan Vanneste and Ron Hyman

Department of Neurology, Sint Lucas Ziekenhuis, Amsterdam, The Netherlands

In a prospective study on normal-pressure hydrocephalus (NPH), CT-cisternography was performed in 17 patients with possible NPH and additional isotope cisternography in 5 of these.

Seventeen patients met the criteria of possible NPH and nine of them, all aged 60 years or over, unexpectedly appeared to have NPH due to non-tumoural aqueduct stenosis. In this subgroup the lateral and third ventricles were markedly dilated, in contrast with a normal fourth ventricle. CT-cisternography was characterized by filling of the fourth ventricle and absence of contrast in the third ventricle, suggesting a block at the level of the aqueduct. Another cause of hydrocephalus could not be demonstrated; we did not find any argument to believe that aqueduct stenosis was secondary to mesencephalic compression by markedly enlarged ventricles, as has been described by B. Williams (Brain 1973; 96: 399–412).

A possible aetiology of aqueduct stenosis was tracable in 6 cases (see *Table*). It was not clear why a so far "silent" hydrocephalus due to aqueduct stenosis became symptomatic in the elderly. Theoretically, further narrowing of the aqueduct by increasing periaqueductal gliosis and subsequent aqueductal incompetence is possible, but this assumption awaits pathological confirmation. Diminished periventricular blood flow may also have been of influence. In conclusion, we found that when in older patients aqueduct stenosis becomes symptomatic, it usually does so in a NPH-fashion, and not in high pressure hydrocephalus, as commonly believed. Our experience suggests that non-tumoural aqueduct stenosis is a common cause of NPH in older patients.   (J Neurol Neurosurg Psychiatry 49: 529–535, 1986)

Key words: Normal-pressure hydrocephalus, Non-communicating hydrocephalus, Aqueduct stenosis, CT-cisternograpy

Table. Clinical data

Patients			History	Duration of symptoms before first examination in years	Signs			Factors aggravating normal pressure hydrocephalus symptoms
No	Sex	Age (yr)			G	M	I	
1	M	68	Severe headache during infancy	5	++	++	−	−
2	M	69	Idem	1	+++	++	Later+	Abdominal surgery
3	F	73	Viral meningoence-phalitis aet. 70 yr	10	++	++	Later+	Mild head injury
4	M	77	—	3	++	+	Later+	Abdominal surgery
5	F	62	Bacterial meningitis aet. 8 yr	4	+	+	−	−
6	F	65	—	5	++	+	Later+	Mild head injury
7	F	72	Head injury aet. 67 yr	5	++	++	−	Head injury
8	M	73	Cytomegaloencephali-tis aet 66 yr?	3	+	+	−	−
9	F	81	—	3	++	+	+	−

Vascular disease	Therapy	Improvement	Further course
Multiple cerebral strokes	VAS	+	Died 2 years later after repeat strokes
Aortic aneurysm peripheral vascular disease	VAS refused, accepted 5 months later after deterioration	++	Died 18 months later from oat-cell carcinoma
Slight hypertension (mean 180/105 mm Hg)	VAS refused, accepted 1 year later after deterioration	++	Improvement persisted for 3 years
—	VAS	++	Improvement persisted until now (4 months)
—	Repeat CSF taps	±	Fluctuating with episodic flare-ups of normal pressure hydrocephalus signs
—	VAS	++	Improvement persisted for 2½ years
—	VAS	—	Further deterioration
—	Repeat CSF taps for 18 months VAS after further deterioration	++	Improvement persisted for 2 years
Minimal hypertension (mean 170/100)	Repeat CSF taps	±	Slight progression of gait instability and mental defects

Abbreviations: G, gait instability; M, mental deterioration; I, incontinence; VAS, ventriculoatrial shunting; (−), absent; (±), fluctuating; (+), slight; (++), moderate; (+++), marked.

Normal Pressure Hydrocephalus: Onset of gait abnormality before dementia predicts good surgical outcome

Neill R. Graff-Radford and John C. Godersky

The University of Iowa, Iowa City, Iowa, IA, USA

In 1977, Fisher reported that in patients with possible normal pressure hydrocephalus (NPH), if the gait abnormality preceded dementia, surgery usually had a favorable outcome and vice versa. We studied this finding in 21 patients shunted for possible NPH. By evaluating serial videotapes of gait, neuropsychological tests and Katz index ratings, preoperatively and at approximately two and six months postoperatively, we judged 16 patients improved. In the improved group, the families reported that the gait abnormality preceded the dementia in 11 patients and occurred at the same time in five. In the unimproved group, dementia was noted first in three patients, gait abnormality first in one patient, and gait and dementia at the same time in one patient. Using Fisher's exact test, we compared the improved and unimproved groups for gait abnormality or dementia onset first and found a significant difference (p=0.0088). Patients with gait onset at the same time as dementia also improved significantly more frequently than those with dementia before gait abnormality (p=0.047), but there were fewer patients in these groups so this result should be treated cautiously. We conclude that the history of gait abnormality occurring before or after dementia in patients with possible NPH is an important prognostic factor for surgical outcome. (Arch Neurol 43: 940–942, 1986)

Key words: Hydrocephalus, Gait, Dementia

Table. Demographic and duration of illness data of patients with normal-pressure hydrocephalus

Patient No./ Age, y/Sex	Improved	Symptom Duration in Years Prior to Surgery		
		Dementia	Gait Abnormality	Incontinence
1/60*/M	Yes	0.50+	0.50+	Urinary urgency
2/79/F	Yes	0.25	0.50+	0.25
3/68/M	Yes	0.50	4.50+	0.25
4/86/M	Yes	0.25	1.00+	0.25
5/69/M	Yes	0.50	1.50+	0.50
6/74/F	Yes	0.75+	0.75+	Urinary urgency
7/72*/M	Yes	2.00	4.00+	2.00
8/73/M	Yes	0.25	2.00+	0.25
9/77/F	Yes	1.00+	1.00+	1.00
10/51/M	Yes	1.00+	1.00+	1.00
11/77/F	Yes	0.25	5.00+	0.25
12/77/F	Yes	1.00	4.00+	0.25
13/73/M	Yes	1.50	2.50+	2.50
14/83/M	Yes	1.00	3.00+	1.50
15/69/M	Yes	0.66+	0.66+	0.33
16/75/F	Yes	1.00	3.00+	0.25
17/82/M	No	4.00	9.00+	4.00
18/76/M	No	1.00+	1.00+	0.50
19/80/M	No	4.00+	0.25	0.25
20/73/M	No	2.00+	1.00	0.26
21/75/M	No	2.50+	0.25	0.25

* Secondary normal-pressure hydrocephalus.
+ First symptom(s) observed.

Normal Pressure Hydrocephalus:
Predictive value of the cerebrospinal fluid tap test

Carsten WIKKELSO,[1] Hugo ANDERSSON,[2] Christian BLOMSTRAND,[1] Göran LINDQVIST,[2] and Pål SVENDSEN[3]

Department of [1]Neurology, [2]Neurosurgery, and [3]Diagnostic Radiology (Neuroradiology), Sahlgren Hospital Gothenburg, Sweden

Twenty-seven patients with normal pressure hydrocephalus were operated upon by a ventriculo-peritoneal shunt. Selection for shunt surgery was based on typical symptoms (gait disturbancy, mental deterioration and urgency incontinence and characteristic changes at cranial computer tomography and/or radionuclide cisternography. Prior to operation a cerebrospinal fluid tap test (CSF-TT) was performed with measurements of psychometric functions and gait pattern before and after a lumbar puncture of 50 cc CSF. Psychometric tests included identical forms measuring complex perceptual functions, Bingley's memory test and reaction time measured as speed of manual reaction to visual or sound stimuli. The walking test was done by counting how many steps a patient needed for walking 18 meters. Mean of 3 tests was calculated.

Neurological and psychiatric examination were registered in semi-quantitative scales. Special attention was paid to symptoms like paratonia, abnormal reflexes and gait pattern. The psychiatric diagnoses used were impairment/off/wakefulness syndrome, astheno-emotional syndrome, emotional/motivational/blunting and Korsakoff's amnesia.

Nineteen patients improved and five were unchanged after shunt operation. Three patients could not be evaluated. Improvement in the psychometric functions and gait pattern after lumbar puncture correlated to improvement after the shunt operation (r=0.64, p<0.01: r=0.96, p<0.001, respectively). Improvement in two or more of the four tests used (3 psychometric and 1 gait test) at CSF-TT implied in all cases successful results of the shunt operation. It was concluded that CSF-TT could predict which NPH patient will improve by a shunt operation and albeit to envisage the degree of improvement. In addition to gait and mental improvement postoperatively, paratonial rigidity and abnormal reflexes (snout) diminished (p<0.05). All patients with impairment/off/wakefulness syndrome before the operation improved. (Acta Neurol Scand 73: 566–573, 1986)

Key words: Normal pressure hydrocephalus, Lumbar puncture, Prediction

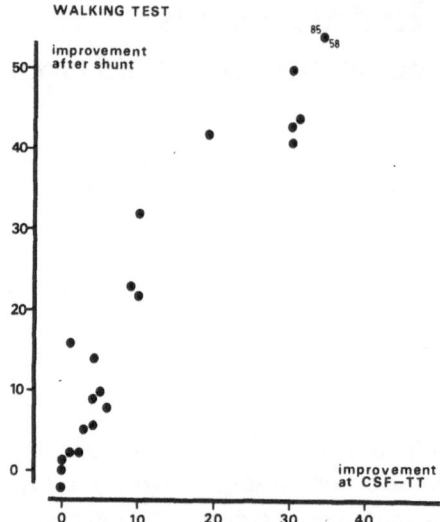

Figure. Improvement in walking pattern (measured as reduction in number of steps needed for walking 18 m) after lumbar puncture (CSF-TT) (abscissa) correlated to improvement after shunt operation (ordinate) measured in the same way. Indicate individual patients. The correlation is significant (r=0.96, p<0.001). The patient indicated in the upper right corner improved 58 steps at CSF-TT and 85 after the operation.

Index

AUTHOR INDEX

SUBJECT INDEX